DE-STRESS, WEIGH LESS

CAN HELP YOU:

- WRITE A STRESS-REDUCTION CONTRACT

- MAKE THE FOOD/STRESS CONNECTION WITH A SIMPLE TEST

- KEEP A FOOD/STRESS DIARY

- STOP BINGE EATING

- DEFINE AND ACHIEVE A STRESS-REDUCTION GOAL

- LEARN HOW SUGAR TRIGGERS STRESS AND WEIGHT GAIN

- DISCOVER HOW B VITAMINS CAN REDUCE YOUR STRESS

. . . AND SO MUCH MORE!

DE-STRESS, WEIGH LESS

PAUL J. ROSCH, M.D., F.A.C.P.
and
CAROLYN CHAMBERS CLARK,
ED.D., R.N., A.R.N.P., F.A.A.N.

St. Martin's Paperbacks

NOTE: If you purchased this book without a cover you should be aware that this book is stolen property. It was reported as "unsold and destroyed" to the publisher, and neither the author nor the publisher has received any payment for this "stripped book."

DE-STRESS, WEIGH LESS

Copyright © 2001 by Paul J. Rosch and Carolyn Chambers Clark.

All rights reserved. No part of this book may be used or reproduced in any manner whatsoever without written permission except in the case of brief quotations embodied in critical articles or reviews. For information address St. Martin's Press, 175 Fifth Avenue, New York, NY 10010.

ISBN: 0-312-97724-7

Printed in the United States of America

St. Martin's Paperbacks edition / June 2001

St. Martin's Paperbacks are published by St. Martin's Press, 175 Fifth Avenue, New York, NY 10010.

10 9 8 7 6 5 4 3 2 1

NOTICE

This book is intended as a reference volume only, not as a medical manual. The information given here is designed to help you make informed decisions about your health. It is not intended as a substitute for any treatment that may have been prescribed by your doctor. If you suspect that you have a medical problem, we urge you to seek competent medical help.

CONTENTS

CONTENTS

DE-STRESS, WEIGH LESS

INTRODUCTION

Why Diets and Diet Pills Won't Work and May Even Harm You

If you're reading this book, chances are that you want to lose weight. Congratulations! You may be about to take a giant step toward health. We'll be right beside you, advising and encouraging you as you work your way toward your goal.

In these pages, you'll learn a fantastic new way to lose weight and keep it off, a way that's not a diet and not a pill. We're not going to tell you that you have to eat only this or that or that you must take a pill every day to lose weight.

HOW THIS BOOK WILL HELP YOU LOSE WEIGHT

Whatever your reason for wanting to lose weight, *De-Stress, Weigh Less* will help. You'll learn how to stop dieting and lose weight permanently. The secret is reducing physiological and psychological stress. It's as simple as reducing your intake of foods when stressed, getting away from binge eating and overzealous exercise programs, and halting other life stressors. We'll show you how, step by step, so that when you're finished reading this book you will not only be losing weight, but you'll also have discovered a prescription for lifelong weight maintenance.

WHO WE ARE AND WHY WE WANTED TO WRITE THIS BOOK

You may want to know more about who we are and why we wanted to write this book. I'm Paul J. Rosch, a medical doctor and president of the American Institute of Stress and clinical professor of medicine and psychiatry at New York Medical College. I studied with Hans Selye, who coined the term *stress*.

I'm Carolyn Chambers Clark, an advanced registered nurse practitioner with a master's degree in mental health nursing and a doctorate in education from Columbia University. I am on the doctoral faculty for the Health Sciences Program at Walden University and have maintained a private wellness education practice for more than thirty years, helping people just like you lose weight and keep it off.

Because we both have an interest in and many years of experience with weight loss, we want to help you learn what you need to know to lose weight and keep it off forever. To help you remember that you are not alone, throughout this book we will be sharing case studies that come from our own practices. Of course, the names and some of the details have been changed, but the basic facts are the same. Join us on this life-changing journey. It may be the best decision you've ever made!

DIETS DON'T WORK AND THEY'RE VERY STRESSFUL

The first stop on our journey together is to take a look at why diets don't work. Does the case study that follows bear any similarity to your situation?

Nancy is a twenty-eight-year-old administrative assistant who always dreamed of fitting into a bikini and looking really good in it. She's tried just about every diet invented, but none of them got her to the size she wanted to be. Sure, she lost a few pounds, some-

times many pounds, but as soon as she stopped dieting the weight always crept back on, until she weighed
even more than she had before she started the diet! In
desperation, Nancy tried a diet pill. Within two weeks,
she had shed ten pounds, but she was so irritable her
friends stopped calling and she couldn't sleep. To her,
it was worth it. Just when Nancy thought she was getting somewhere, she developed high blood pressure
and constant diarrhea from the diet pills. It was then
she decided to try a safer and healthier way of losing
weight and began the plan found in this book.

Despite your thinking that the latest "crash diet" will do it
for you, there is solid research that shows it won't. Recent
research reported in *Obesity Research*[1] found that frequent dieters showed significantly more weight regain
than less frequent dieters. Research published in the
Journal of Consulting Clinical Psychology in 1999[2]
found that even among young girls, those who "dieted"
were more likely to weigh more and that obesity was
strongly associated with attempts to control weight. Each
increase in appetite suppressant and laxative use was reflected in an 85 percent increased risk of obesity. These
researchers concluded that weight-reducing efforts can
lead to dysregulation of the normal appetite system, resulting in weight gain from erratic eating behaviors and
decreased metabolism efficiency.

We know how easy it is to latch on to some new fad
diet or diet pill in the hope that "this will be the one that
works!" None of them do—at least not for long—and you
do run the risk of nasty side effects.

WHY DIETS CAN HURT YOU

The low-carbohydrate, high-protein diet that is currently
in vogue is hardly new but is just a resurrection of the regimen introduced two decades ago, which goes back to the
Civil War era, when it was proposed by William Banting,

a London undertaker. It has also periodically resurfaced as the Pennington, Canadian Air Force, Calories Don't Count, Drinking Man's, Stilman, and Scarsdale Diets. Each of these diets allow you to stuff yourself with all the ice cream, eggs, and meat you want. It's fun at first, but very quickly it becomes a boring way to eat and makes you feel awful.

But the real concern is that high-protein diets may also be unhealthy because they don't contain enough nutrients to keep you healthy or to help your body processes work efficiently so you can take weight off and keep it off.[3, 4] Also, researchers warn that by limiting what you eat you may cause yourself to have significantly less bone mineral density and less bone mineral content than if you eat healthily.[5, 6] The ketones that accumulate when you eat too much protein and fat can also be damaging to your kidneys and give you headaches and bad breath and even make you feel dizzy. Because these diets don't contain enough fiber, they can also lead to constipation.

Even more frightening, the high saturated fat content allowed in these diets is one of the major risk factors for heart attacks, strokes, and certain cancers. Worse, you will increase your risk for cancer and heart disease even more because you will be restricting the very foods that research has shown will protect you from these conditions—vegetables, fruits, and grains.[7]

The proponents of these diets claim they are safe, but we cannot agree. For your best health and weight loss, stay away from these and other fad diets—they aren't healthy and, for long-term weight loss, they just don't work.

The fact is no diet works and "yo-yo" dieting or weight cycling, where weight is quickly lost and then gained back again, is very stressful.[7] This kind of temporary weight loss can increase the risk of gallstones and boosts the need for gallbladder surgery. A study published in a 1999 issue of the *Annals of Internal Medicine*[8] showed that women with moderate weight fluctuations (ten- to nineteen-pound weight loss) had a 31 percent greater risk of gallstones and gallbladder surgery, while women with severe weight cycling (twenty-pound or more weight loss) had a 68 percent greater risk.

Weight cycling is also bad for the heart. Although there may be some benefits from the effects of losing weight, these benefits are quickly offset by the rebound phenomenon that occurs when weight is regained, including increased blood pressure, disturbances in heart rhythm, and defects in heart function and blood pressure. Weight cycling tends to redistribute fat to the abdomen, and the resulting increased waist:hip ratio is a factor for risk of heart attack. Recent research confirms that repeated dieting for weight loss increases deaths due to cardiovascular causes.[7] In fact, a 1992 study in the *Journal of the American Medical Association*[9] showed that yo-yo dieting and its resultant weight fluctuation increased death rates by more than 50 percent.

Dieting can also be stressful for your body, because it can lead to eating fewer sources of natural antioxidants that fight the free radicals that can cause cellular damage. Excess free radicals are found in pesticides, acid rain, artificial preservatives and additives, and a whole host of environmental pollutants. Just taking a vitamin pill isn't going to provide the antioxidant protection that fresh fruits and vegetables do. Research has shown that these foods contain other substances that potentiate protection from free radicals.[10, 11] For some reason, yet unknown, eating a small amount of foods rich in antioxidants can protect you much better than thousands of units of a vitamin.

HOW DIETING PUTS ON WEIGHT AND HURTS YOU IN OTHER WAYS

Dieting leads to the "Dieter's Dilemma," a term fir[-] coined by William Bennett at Harvard University. [-]

dilemma proceeds as follows: due to a desire to be thin, eating is restricted; this results in cravings and reduced self-control, which leads to a loss of control and overeating, which in turn leads to regained weight and a need to repeat the cycle. Again, diets actually cause weight gain, not weight loss.

The results of a University of Toronto study, published in the *International Journal of Eating Disorders*,[12] found that dieting leads to false hope that fuels dieter attempts on one diet after another even through failure and depression because the new diet that doesn't work is just around the corner. Think back to your dieting experiences. At first, you may have gotten a rush of hope at the thought of a new diet. You may have even felt hopeful of your potential success but also more depressed, thinking, *Here I go again. This diet is never going to work.* Guess what? It's not.

Dieting is also harmful because it leads to binge eating and is correlated with dangerous medical conditions such as bulimia. As tension builds from feeling deprived while dieting, binge eating steps in. A study published in a 1999 issue of the *Journal of Eating Disorders*[13] found that the women most apt to binge were the ones who had been on one or more diets in the past year. The more these women tried to restrict their food, the more they binged and exercised excessively and the more likely they were to be bulimic. Even if bulimia was not reported, women who binged were also more likely to drop out of weight management programs, possibly making them feel even more desperate and like more of a failure. Research published in a 1997 issue of the *International Journal of Eating Disorders*[14] found that despite ethnic background, binge eaters reported going on more diets and having more restrictive attitudes about their weight and shape and higher levels of depression.

Dieting can also make you feel dopey, irritable, and tired, and can slow your reaction speed and mental performance. This research, published in a 1998 issue of the *Journal of Clinical Psychology*,[15] found that participants on diets invariably had reaction and mental performance deficits comparable to those caused by having had two alcoholic drinks. The culprit was not the lower caloric intake but the stress of dieting. The ones who did the worst on the performance tests were on diets and weren't losing weight. So not only do diets not work and put unhealthy stress on your body, but the emotional stress of constantly worrying about what to eat can also impair your mental performance. Instead of going on yet another diet that can make you feel terrible and ensure that you will regain any weight you do lose, read on.

BUT WHAT ABOUT WEIGHT LOSS DRUGS?

Diet drugs don't work, either. Some amphetamines, such as Benzedrine and Dexedrine, have been banned because they can cause excess stimulation and addiction. Phenylpropanol amine, a common ingredient of nonprescription cold and weight loss medicines (Dexatrim, Acutrim) was just banned because of stroke risk. Sales of fenfluramine, a serotonin booster, exploded a few years ago when it was reported to be safe and effective. It was withdrawn from the market when serious—even fatal—side effects occurred. Since then, numerous weight loss pills have been developed and approved, but none of them has been proven effective for the long term and all cause problems and have side effects that range from annoying to serious. Even herbal weight loss products, such as Metabolife, have not been tested for their long-term weight loss effectiveness and undesirable effects.

It's only human nature to want a magic bullet that will take away the fat and keep it off, but that just isn't possible. So read on! *De-Stress, Weigh Less* will give you a doable alternative to dieting that uses approaches that are safe and that work.

REFERENCES

1. Pasman, W. J., W. H. Saris, and M. S. Westerterp-Plantenga. 1999. Predictors of weight maintenance. *Obesity Research* 7(1): 43–50.

2. Stice, E., R. P. Cameron, and C. Hayward. 1999. Naturalistic weight-reduction efforts prospectively predict growth in relative weight and onset of obesity among female adolescents. *Journal of Consulting Clinical Psychology* 67: 967–74.

3. Zemel, M. B., H. Shi, B. Greer, D. Dirienzo, and P. C. Zemel. 2000. Regulation of adiposity by dietary calcium. *FASEB J* 14(9): 1132–38.

4. Al Zahrani, H., R. W. Norman, C. Thompson, and S. Weerasinghe 2000. The dietary habits of calcium stone-formers and normal control subjects. *BJU International* 85(6): 616–20.

5. Hannan, M. T., D. T. Felson, B. Dawson-Hughes, K. L. Tucker, L. A. Cupples, P. W. Wilson, and D. P. Kiel. 2000. Risk factors for longitudinal bone loss in elderly men and women: The Framingham Osteoporosis Study. *Journal of Bone Mineral Research* 15(4): 710–20.

6. Gossain, V. V., D. S. Rao, M. J. Carella, G. Divine, and D. R. Rovner. 1999. Bone mineral density (BMD) in obesity effect of weight loss. *Journal of Medicine* 30(5–6): 367–76.

7. Rosch, P. 1993. Yo-yo dieting and coronaries. *Health and Stress* 4: 7.

8. Syngal, S., E. H. Coakley, W. C. Willett, T. Byers, D. F. Williamson, and G. A. Colditz. 1999. Long-term weight patterns and risk for cholecystectomy in women. *Annals of Internal Medicine* 130(6): 471–77.

9. Lee, I. M., and R. S. Paffenbarger. 1992. Change in body weight and longevity. *Journal of the American Medical Association* 268(15): 2045–49.

10. Halliwell, B. 1993. The role of oxygen radicals in human disease, with particular reference to the vascular system. *Haemostasis* 23(Supplement 1): 118–26.

11. Milner J. A. 1986. Dietary antioxidants and cancer. *ASDC J Dent Child* 53(2):140–43.

12. Polivy, J., and C. P. Herman. 1999. The effects of resolving

to diet on restrained and unrestrained eaters: The "false hope syndrome." *International Journal of Eating Disorders* 26(4): 434–37.

13. Kinzl, J. F., C. Traweger, E. Trefalt, B. Mangweth, and W. Biebl. 1999. Binge eating disorder in females: A population-based investigation. *Journal of Eating Disorders* 25(3): 287–92.

14. French, S. A., M. Story, D. Neumark-Sztainer, B. Downes, M. Resnick, and R. Blum. 1997. Ethnic differences in psychosocial and health behavior correlates of dieting, purging, and binge eating in a population-based sample of adolescent females. *International Journal of Eating Disorders* 22(3): 315–322.

15. Hart, K. E., and P. Chiovari. 1998. Inhibition of eating behavior: Negative cognitive effects of dieting. *Journal of Clinical Psychology* 54(4): 427–30.

CHAPTER 1

How Stress Plays a Role in Weight Gain

Numerous studies show that 95 percent of all individuals who do manage to lose weight will gain it back again in three to five years (or sooner), usually putting on more weight than they lost. We believe, and the research shows, that stress plays a major role in weight gain.

WHAT IS STRESS AND HOW DOES IT AFFECT YOU?

According to Hans Selye, the father of the term, stress is normal wear and tear on the body due to internal and external events.[1] But what most people often think of as "stress" is actually what William Cannon described in 1914[2] as the fight or flight response, an emergency reaction that prepares you to fight or run. Physiological changes you experience in this response include an increase in blood pressure, heart rate, breathing, metabolism, adrenaline, cortisol, and blood glucose (sugar); shunting of blood away from the gut to the large muscles of the extremities to provide greater strength for "fight or flight." This was useful and life-saving for primitive man suddenly faced with a predator. But now, when you get all worked up and don't run it off, stress builds up in your tissues. Over time, chronic stress weakens your immune system, lowering resistance to infections and viral-linked disorders, including cancer.[3]

Not all stress is negative, but too much of it certainly is. Stress has been related to many diseases and ailments, including headaches, peptic ulcers, arthritis, colitis, diarrhea, asthma, cardiac arrhythmias, sexual problems, circulation problems, muscle tension, and cancer.[3] Numerous studies[4,5,6,7,8,9,10] show that too much stress can result in overeating, eating too quickly, worrying about eating, and eating the wrong foods.

STRESS CAN AFFECT YOUR EATING PATTERNS

Perhaps the most important factor that contributes to unsuccessful weight loss is a lack of understanding about how stress is causing weight gain and regain. One reason for this is that stressed eating leads to eating quickly and binging, because the chemical messengers that influence why, what, when, and how much is eaten (including serotonin, dopamine, noradrenaline, endorphins, and melatonin) function less effectively in a stress condition, making it impossible to tell when you have eaten enough.[11,12,13] Eventually, if you are under continual stress, you will not even pay attention to these signals and they fade from your consciousness. When stress, not hunger, drives eating, overeating results, making it impossible to get to and stay at a healthy weight.

Another stressful behavior that can lead to becoming overweight is night eating.[14] There is some evidence that late night eating inhibits dreaming. This occurs during REM sleep, which is largely responsible for the restorative properties of a good night's rest. Food cannot be digested properly or burned through daily activity and usually ends up as body fat. Thus, night eating can lead to higher stress levels, which will perpetuate this vicious cycle.

More importantly, calories consumed at night tend to be stored as fat since they are usually not burned up by physical activities. Primitive man led a hunter-gatherer existence for millennia and ate whenever food was available, especially if it were meat or something that would spoil. There was no breakfast, lunch, and supper, and one meal a day was more likely the rule. During extended periods of deprivation or starvation, mechanisms designed to reduce caloric expenditure were set into motion and energy came from fat stores. Those who could do this more efficiently were the ones most likely to survive and pass these traits along to future generations. As with certain "fight or flight" reactions that were also once life saving, this metabolic response may have now boomeranged.

When you get up in the morning, you may have had nothing to eat for twelve hours. If you skip breakfast or just have a cup of coffee you may for practical purposes starve for another four or five hours. As far as the body is concerned, this is a signal that you need to conserve calories to survive and it does everything it can to insure this. If you have dinner at seven or later your body believes that you need energy to fight some battle and gears itself for this purpose. But what usually happens is that instead of engaging in any physical activity, you plop down in a chair to watch TV for several hours, and then go to bed. All the calories from dinner poised to be used for work are therefore diverted to fat depots in the body and stored for future use.

While in high school, I (Dr. Rosch) spent my summers working on a farm in Vermont as part of a program to help replace workers drafted during World War II. The farmers got up around 6 A.M., had a huge breakfast of eggs, bacon, pancakes with syrup, bread lathered with butter, and sweet buns, a modest lunch at noon, a sparse dinner at 5 P.M., and generally retired early. Although they probably consumed over 3000 calories a day, I don't recall any that were obese or even significantly overweight.

During the late 1950's, the Army had a crackdown on obesity. While physical requirements were fairly strict on entry, many senior officers were no longer fit for fighting a decade or so later. Those who were grossly overweight were ordered to correct the problem by the time of their next annual physical if they wanted to avoid being discharged. The results were disappointing. Many insisted that although they had faithfully followed their weight reduction diets for several months they had lost only a pound or two, if any, and had actually gained. In a few who had been hospitalized for other reasons and placed on a 1000-calorie diet, hospital records seemed to support their stories.

I was in charge of the Endocrine section of the Department of Metabolism at Walter Reed at the time. Since it was impossible to rule out the possibility that some hormonal disturbance was the cause of their problem or that they were cheating, some of the most stubborn or suspicious cases were admitted to our Metabolic Ward 38 for further investigation and observation. All were placed under constant surveillance and everything they consumed on their 1000-calorie diet was carefully measured and analyzed. They also received a thorough physical examination and an extensive endocrine and metabolic workup to rule out any thyroid or other hormonal disturbance. While regular exercise was encouraged it was not mandated and physical activity and water intake were the only relevant variables.

After one month, sure enough, more of our "prisoners" failed to demonstrate any appreciable weight loss, although those who exercised fared a little better. Nobody knew anything about set points at the time, but I do recall that many had a family history of obesity. Remembering my experience with the farmers, I gave a few patients the same amount of food, but substituted dinner for breakfast. Without any change in total daily caloric intake, some now began to lose weight.

What intrigued me when I later entered private practice was that almost every obese patient I saw would invariably say "I don't understand it, Doctor. I hardly eat anything for breakfast or lunch." This was usually supported by the food diaries I asked them to keep confirming that they should have lost weight based on the total number of calories consumed daily for the past two weeks. I would tell them about my experiences in Vermont and at Walter Reed and urge them to try to eat more for breakfast and less for supper, to eat as early as possible in the evening and try to take a brisk walk afterwards. It was very difficult for more to change their ingrained habits, but those who did stopped gaining weight and started to lose.

These results were recently replicated in a report revealing that eating light all day but having a large evening meal makes you store fat more readily. The subjects in this study were young, elite female athletes, not corpulent Army colonels. Despite reduced total daily caloric intake and very vigorous daily physical exercise, they showed little or no weight loss and their fat deposits increased.

So, if you want to lose weight, in addition to reducing caloric intake, it would be wise to remember the old adage "Eat breakfast like a king, lunch like a prince, and dinner like a pauper."

Dieting can actually *increase* stress and lead to binging. When you feel deprived because your diet is restricted, obsessive thoughts of eating and food take over. Feelings of dissatisfaction, failure, eroded sense of trust in self regarding food choices, and depression can result.[4,5,7,8]

THE RESEARCH SHOWS STRESS LEADS TO WEIGHT GAIN

A 1999 survey published in *Physiological Behavior*[11] found that the majority of its respondents reported that stress levels affected the overall amount of food they ate, with dieters being far more likely to report stress-related binging. Snacking behavior was reportedly increased by stress in the majority of participants (73 percent) regardless of gender. The overall increase in snacking during stress was reflected in their reports of increased intake of "snack-type" foods. In contrast, "meal-type" foods (fruit, vegetables, meat, and fish) were reported to decrease during stressful periods. What the results of this show is that the very people (the stressed-out respondents) who most need the wholesome foods that can reduce stress and increase energy are the very ones who eat "snack" foods, many of which have too much fat and sugar, which can increase stress and lead to weight gain.

There are numerous examples of how stress can lead to weight gain and even obesity, which has become a major problem. Over 70 percent of adult Americans are now considered to be overweight compared to around 55 percent twenty-five years ago. It is no coincidence that surveys show that stress levels have also risen progressively and to the same proportion over this identical period of time. Many people tend to eat more when they are under stress, and usually the wrong things, like sweets and fast foods. Others turn to alcohol, which is another contributor to obesity and a "beer belly." Obesity in children and teens has also reached epidemic proportions and according to a recent Harvard report is now the leading pediatric health problem in the U.S. The prevalence of obesity in children increased by 100 percent between 1980 and 1994 and is still rising. Kids tend to reach for sweets when they are under stress, especially soft drinks. In the last 10 years, soft drink consumption about doubled for children. The average teenager consumes 15 to 20 extra teaspoons of sugar a day from soda and other sugared drinks, many of which tend to be addictive because they contain caffeine. The Harvard study found that adding just one liquid candy drink a day puts a child at 60 percent greater risk for obesity.

One common example of how stress leads to being overweight is the so-called "Freshman Fifteen." This refers to the well documented observation that during the first year of college, the average freshman gains around 15 lbs. One study found that a sample of university women gained weight 36 times faster than controls the same age who did not attend college. Many teenagers move out of their parents' home for the first time, some move out of state, the stress buffering social support provided by family and friends may no longer be available, and all have to adjust to new peers and teachers. The stress of such changes causes many to turn to food for comfort. Food is also used to socialize and make new friends. Pizza parties with soda or beer, midnight vending machine raids, and various food-oriented activities are convenient ways to develop a feeling of belonging and community that helps to reduce stress. Unfortunately, this type of eating either alone or in groups is usually done in addition to regular meals. Freshmen also often eat in a campus cafeteria where they are apt to have a meal plan that offers unlimited buffet-style food, including desserts. This has been described as a "stress test for binge eating" by the Director of the Johns Hopkins Weight Management Center.

Another illustration is "middle-age spread." Many people find that chocolates, cookies, candies, chips, or other high-fat, high-carbohydrate foods seem to relieve their stress. It should be emphasized that the most prominent and important hormonal effect of chronic stress is an increase in cortisol levels. Because of cortisol, these extra calories tend to be stored in fat depots deep in the abdomen, especially in females. The reason is that abdominal fat cells have many more receptors for cortisol than any other part of the body. Cortisol is preferentially attracted to these sites so that the liver can have close and quick access to fuel that might be needed to support physical activities. Cushing's syndrome, which is due to high cortisol levels, is characterized by a marked increase in abdominal obesity. In patients where the disorder is due to a pituitary tumor, this central obesity diminishes or even disappears following removal of the lesion. Further support comes from a study of Swedish men showing that those with the highest levels of chronic stress also had the highest levels of cortisol and the greatest amount of deep-belly fat. In laboratory studies of chronically stressed primates, those having higher cortisol levels similarly showed the highest increases in abdominal fat.

Middle-age spread is a particular problem for women. Female hormones that normally protect against abdominal fat buildup fall dramatically following menopause, eventually resulting in an apple shaped figure. According to Pamela Peeke, a former senior scientist at the National Institutes of Health and Associate Professor of Medicine at the University of Maryland School of Medicine, "It's not just what you weigh; it's where you weigh it. When most women hit 40, they discover that their once-shapely figures have gone from an hourglass to a shot glass." In her recent book *Fight Fat After Forty,* she refers to this as the "menopot."

In addition to being unsightly, an apple shaped figure has been shown to be associated with increased risk for heart disease, stroke, diabetes, and certain cancers. You will find other examples of how stress can lead to eating habits that impair health in subsequent chapters. Based on these and numerous other studies, it is clear that stress reduction is crucial to losing those extra pounds, and more importantly, keeping them off. That's why popular diet plans like Weight Watchers and Jenny Craig now include stress reduction as a crucial component of their programs. So let's start the *De-Stress* Plan, which will allow you to obtain not only maximal benefits for weight loss, but also improved mental and physical health.[15, 16]

REFERENCES

1. Selye, H. 1956. *The Stress of Life*. New York: McGraw-Hill.

2. Cannon, W. 1914. The emergency function of the medulla in pain and the major emotions. *American Journal of Physiology* 33: 356–72.

3. Rosch, R. J. 1996. Stress and Cancer: disorders of communication, control and civilization. In *Handbook of Stress, Medicine and Health*. C. L. Cooper ed., Boca Raton: CRC Press.

4. Stein, K. F., and K. M. Hedger. 1997. Body weight and shape self-cognitions, emotional distress, and disordered eating in middle adolescent girls. *Archives of Psychiatric Nursing* 11(5): 264–75.

5. Polivy, J., and C. P. Herman. 1999. The effects of resolving to diet on restrained and unrestrained eaters: The "false hope syndrome." *International Journal of Eating Disorders* 26(4): 434–37.

6. Ponto, M. 1995. The relationship between obesity, dieting and eating disorders. *Professional Nurse* 10(7): 422–25.

7. Popkess-Vawter, S., S. Wendel, S. Schmoll, and K. O'Connell. 1998. Overeating, reversal theory, and weight cycling. *Western Journal of Nursing Research* 20(1): 67–83.

8. Rozin, P., C. Fischler, S. Imada, A. Sarubin, and A. Wrzesniewski. 1999. Attitudes to food and the role of food in life in the U.S.A., Japan, Flemish Belgium and France: Possible implications for the diet-health debate. *Appetite* 33(2): 163–80.

9. Kinzl, J. F., C. Traweger, E. Trefalt, B. Mangweth, and W. Biebl. 1999. Binge eating disorder in females: A population-based investigation. *Journal of Eating Disorders* 25(3): 287–92.

10. Hart, K. E., and P. Chiovari. 1998. Inhibition of eating behavior: Negative cognitive effects of dieting. *Journal of Clinical Psychology* 54(4): 427–30.

11. Oliver, G., and J. Wardel. 1999. Perceived effects of stress on food choice. *Physiological Behavior* 66 (3): 511–13.

12. Pasman, W. J., W. H. Saris, and M. S. Westerterp-Plantenga. 1999. Predictors of weight maintenance. *Obesity Research* 7(1): 43–50.

13. Thorburn, A. W., and J. Proietto. 1998. Neuropeptides, the hypothalamus and obesity: Insights into the central control of body weight. *Pathology* 30(3): 229–36.

14. Adami, G. F., A. Meneghelli, and N. Scopinaro. 1999. Night eating and binge eating disorder in obese patients. *International Journal of Eating Disorders* 25(3): 335–38.

15. Ludwig, D. S., Peterson, K. E. and Gortmaker, S. L. 2001. Relation between consumption of sugar-sweetened drinks and childhood obesity: a prospective, observational analysis, *Lancet,* 357: 505–08.

16. Peeke, P. 2000. *Fight Fat After Forty: The Revolutionary Three-Pronged Approach That Will Break Your Stress-Fat Cycle and Make You Healthy, Fit, and Trim for Life,* New York: Viking Press.

CHAPTER 2

Step 1: Discover How Stress Is Keeping You Overweight

The term *set point* refers to the weight at which the body stops losing weight because a starvation condition registers. According to the theory, the body does not know the difference between dieting and starvation, so to conserve sufficient energy to keep the body functioning, it shifts into a starvation mode, requiring fewer calories to do the work of the body's metabolic processes. This makes weight loss by severely restricting food and calories nearly impossible. Although set points are believed to be genetically determined, it may be possible to reset them through slow and steady weight loss.[1]

CREATING A PERSONALIZED WEIGHT LOSS PLAN

Over time, the chronic stress of dieting leads not only to weight gain but also to actual physiological changes in your body. Fortunately, most of this can be reversed with healthy, stress-reducing behaviors. The rest of this book provides the tools for reducing stress. The first step to take is to identify your sources of stress so you can create a personal weight loss plan.

Because no one approach works for everyone, this book is about alternatives. Information will be provided to help you choose an approach that will work for you. Specific suggestions for how to stick with the chosen method are provided, along with positive ideas for implementing action.

DEVELOP A CONTRACT TO GET YOURSELF GOING

A contract is an effective way to get you started in the direction of taking charge and losing weight healthily. Read and fill in the contract provided here. If you like, change the wording to suit you. The idea is to identify a specific goal to work on and then take active steps to meet that goal. The more you set specific goals, work toward them, and reward yourself, the more successful you'll be. If you have a general goal, like reading this book, it could seem overwhelming, but if you break it down into small steps, like reading a chapter a day or trying out one new stress-reduction idea each day, it's much easier.

Find a concerned significant other in your life to cosign the contract and promise to help you follow through on your commitment. That not only will provide you with support for your weight loss activities but can also keep you focused. Be sure to choose someone who won't nag you or be negative. We suggest that you find a positive, supportive person, because the research shows that such a person can help you lose the weight you want to lose.

I, _____ [your name], agree to read a chapter of this book a day and try out at least one idea from each chapter.

SIGNED _____ DATE _____

COSIGNED _____ DATE _____
I will reward myself for reading each chapter or trying out a new stress-reduction idea by:

_____

Be sure to reward yourself once you've completed each task. If you usually use food as your reward, think about trying something different, like watching a movie you'd like to see, getting a back rub or massage, going to a concert or museum, or just treating yourself nicely in some other way.

HOW STRESS MAY BE KEEPING YOU OVERWEIGHT

Before you take a look at how stress is keeping you overweight, let's discuss John, a hypothetical case based on many individuals we've seen who wanted to lose weight.

> John is a twenty-year-old college student. His father wants him to be a doctor, but he is having trouble with organic chemistry and most of the other courses he had to take. He's been overweight off and on since grade school, and his mother sometimes teases him about his weight. As a result, he tries every new diet that comes around. He's been eating a high-protein diet for the past two weeks but has been bothered by feelings of dizziness. Although he's not supposed to eat sweets, when he studies he sometimes takes a few of his roommate's cookies or candy bars, telling himself, "A little of this can't hurt." Although he's been on many diets, he always gains back what he loses, plus ten or more pounds. He hopes he doesn't end up like his uncle who was overweight and died of a heart attack.

Let's take a look at how stress is keeping John overweight. His father's expectations are certainly one source of stress, but what about his mother's teasing? Having trouble in school and yo-yo dieting are other things that stress him. As we mentioned in chapter 1, the high-protein diet he's on is stressful, too, as evidenced by his dizziness. John starts to binge and of course he picks the very foods he's supposed to be restricting, possibly because he feels deprived by not being able to eat those foods. The binging indicates he's lost his ability to tune into his own hunger signals, another sign of stress. Finally, he is driven to eat because he's afraid of having a heart attack and repeating what happened to his uncle. What John doesn't know yet is that the foods he's eating and the way he's acting are the stressful things that could lead to a heart attack. Too bad John didn't take the Stress Test you're going to have an opportunity to take in just a minute. Taking the Stress Test may just prevent you from repeating John's mistakes.

FIND OUT WHAT STRESS MAY BE KEEPING YOU OVERWEIGHT

Once you identify changes in your life that are producing stress, you can move onto specific ways to relax and keep weight off.

By now, you're beginning to get a pretty good idea of how stress is affecting your mind, body, and spirit. Now's the time to think about how each change and each stress symptom you have may be related to your eating patterns. To begin that process, ask yourself these questions:

1. Did I gain weight after something in my work or school changed?
2. Did I gain weight after I lost someone or something very important to me?
3. Did I gain weight after I moved to a new home?
4. Did I gain weight after my life changed?
5. Did I gain weight after I made (or lost) a specific amount of money?
6. Did I gain weight after a specific challenge I had to adjust to?
7. Did I gain weight after I started worrying more about things?
8. Do I eat before, after, or during the time I feel anxious about being tested or evaluated?

9. Do I eat before, after, or during the time I feel anxious about making deadlines?
10. Do I eat before, after, or during the time I feel anxious about being interviewed?
11. Do I eat before, after, or during the time I feel anxious about performing (physically, sexually, mentally, emotionally, or spiritually)?
12. Do I eat before, during, or after the time I feel anxious in personal relationships with a partner, a date, parents, children, friends, strangers, or others?
13. Do I eat when I feel depressed?
14. Do I eat when I feel hopeless?
15. Do I eat when I feel powerless?
16. Do I eat when I feel bad about myself?
17. Do I eat when I feel hostile or when others are hostile toward me?
18. Do I eat when I feel resentful?
19. Do I eat when I feel angry or others show anger with me?
20. Do I eat when I feel irritable or when others are irritated with me?
21. Do I eat when I'm afraid of something?
22. Do I eat when I'm bothered by unwanted thoughts?
23. Do I eat because I have high blood pressure?
24. Do I eat when I have a headache or to ward one off?
25. Do I eat when my neck aches?
26. Do I eat when I have a backache?
27. Do I eat until I have indigestion?
28. Do I eat until my stomach/lower bowel makes weird noises and messes up my bowel movements?
29. Do I eat when my stomach burns?
30. Do I eat when I'm constipated?
31. Do I eat when I'm feeling fatigued?

32. Do I eat when I can't sleep?
33. Do I eat because I'm overweight?
34. Did I start eating more once I was diagnosed with an illness/condition?

If the answer to any of these is yes, congratulations. You are beginning to make connections between what happens in your life to stress you and your eating patterns. As you make more and more connections, you will begin to see which stresses you will be most likely able to control or change for the better. In chapters 5 and 7, we will help you find the best stress management techniques for the situations that cause you the most anxiety. For now, remember this information or put a paper clip on this page so you can refer back to it.

Chart Your Food and Mood

Stress has a great effect on what you eat, when, how much you eat, and whether you enjoy it or not. You may not believe it—or maybe you do because you do the same thing—but many overweight people do not get much enjoyment out of the food they eat. Sometimes they don't even taste it because they're eating too fast or thinking about something else. Sometimes they don't enjoy their food because they're feeling guilty because they're eating foods they don't think they should be eating.

By keeping a Food/Stress Diary (for at least a week) of the time you eat and what you thought and did while eating, you can begin to see stress patterns that can keep you overeating and overweight. By keeping this diary, you will begin to see the patterns in your eating behavior. Finding patterns is the first step toward getting control over your weight. As you use the Food/Stress Diary for the next week, remember that you are a unique person with unique reactions to food and stress. You will begin to see just how much of what you eat and why is a reaction to stress, not hunger. That is a very important step toward keeping weight off. Once you begin to see how food and stress interact in your life, you can begin to take charge.

Make enough copies of the Food/Stress Diary to last for a week. A page or two should do you for each day. Look for your eating patterns. Here are some questions to get you started:

- Do you always reach for chocolate, French fries, or some other favorite food when you are feeling upset?
- Do you keep "goodies" in your desk drawer to pop in your mouth when you feel stressed?
- Do you open the freezer and eat half a gallon of ice cream after a rough day at work or school?
- Do you stop for a hamburger and fries after a bad day at work?
- Do you stop for fried chicken because it's close by and you forgot your lunch?

You get the idea. Now make up your own questions about stress and food and see what you can find out.

There are as many food/stress patterns as there are people. See how your stress is causing you to overeat or eat the wrong kinds of foods. In the chapters that follow, you'll find out which foods may be adding to your stress, thus keeping your weight on. You'll also find out which foods create less stress for you. Later on, you'll learn how to retrain your stress response so you can stop binging, combine food and exercise to reduce stress and reduce other life stressors that may be keeping you from losing weight. There is one more piece to discovering how stress is keeping you overweight. That piece will be found in your answers to the Food/Stress Diary.

THE FOOD/STRESS DIARY[3]
Fill out the following form every day for a week to examine how food may be stressing you. Try to make an entry

every time you eat something, even if it's "only a taste" of someone else's brownie or ice-cream cone. Try to be as honest as you can. Remember, nobody's watching. This is only to help you take charge of your weight. Look at the sample entries, and then fill in your own.

FOOD/STRESS DIARY					
DAY/TIME	EVENT	REACTIONS	HUNGER*	FOOD	THOUGHTS/ FEELINGS
Monday, 8:00 A.M.	job evaluation today	stomach hurts	1	pie	thinking about my boss
Monday, 10:00 A.M.	indigestion	I shouldn't have had that pie	1	coffee	I'm not eating 'til dinner!
Monday, 1:00 P.M.	bad job evaluation	I'm a failure	2	ice cream	I deserve better than this

Your turn:

_____

_____

_____

*FROM 1 (LITTLE HUNGER) TO 10 (STARVING)

After you've completed your Food/Stress Diary for a week, take a look at all the pages. What patterns do you notice? Which days and times of the day are you most apt to eat when you feel stressed? Are you always hungry when you eat or do you eat when you are just stressed? What are you most likely to eat when you feel stressed? Which foods seem most connected to your stress symptoms?

CHOOSE A STRESS-REDUCTION GOAL YOU CAN LIVE WITH

Now that you've completed the Food/Stress Diary, it's time to choose a stress-reduction goal. Look at the following list of alternatives, pick the one that makes the most sense to you, and place a check in front of it. Make your choice based on what feels comfortable for you now. Maybe you're ready to start shaping what you eat to reduce your stress. Or maybe you're more ready to start an exercise program or stop binging. You may even be ready to tackle those other stresses in your life that make you want to gobble food every time you think about them. It doesn't matter; just take the time to choose a goal.

CHOOSING A STRESS-REDUCTION GOAL

DIRECTIONS: Place a check in front of one of the following goals. Choose one that most appeals to you, then go right to the suggested chapter for ideas about how to meet that goal. When you've reached that goal, come back to this table and choose your next goal. You may decide to use the same goal but change the food or learn another stress-reduction skill. That's OK. Your choice. Eventually you will work your way through all six steps. Remember to take your time and move at your own pace. We want you to feel comfortable and in charge.

Stress-Reduction Goals

____ Stop eating in ways that may be stressful (see chapter 3 for ideas)

____ Start eating more healthily (see chapter 4 for ideas)

____ Take one action to train myself to stop binging (see chapter 5 for ideas)

____ Start a stress-*less* exercise program (see chapter 6 for ideas)

___ Use one stress-reduction skill to reduce my life stressors
that are keeping me from losing weight (see chapter 7 for
ideas)

Whichever one you choose is right for you now. Begin
to work on that goal now. There is no right order for
working in this book or for reducing stress. You can skip
ahead to other chapters based on what is important to you
right this moment. Remember, we'll be with you no matter which path you choose, cheering you on, knowing you
can do this, and telling you that all it takes is a little effort
and persistence.

REFERENCES
1. Thorburn, A. W., and J. Proietto. 1998. Neuropeptides, the
   hypothalamus and obesity: Insights into the central control
   of body weight. *Pathology* 30(3): 229–36.
2. Miller, M. A., and R. H. Rahe. 1997. Life Changes Scaling
   for the 1990s. *Journal of Psychosomatic Research* 43(3):
   279–92.
3. Clark, C. C. 1996. *Wellness Practitioner: Concepts, Research and Strategies*. New York: Springer.

CHAPTER 3

Step 2: Eliminate Foods That May Be Stressing You

Because everyone is unique, some of the foods we discuss in this chapter may be stressful for you, while others may not be. Try to identify and eliminate foods that may be stressful and could be interfering with your plans to lose weight. First, let's take a look at what and how Emily eats that could be stressing her and leading to weight problems.

Emily is a forty-year-old software programmer who loves chocolate. She eats brownies, drinks colas, and has a couple of candy bars every day. Emily can't wait for her break so she can enjoy her cola and candy bar. She quickly eats the candy bar, barely tasting it, and washes it down with the soda. She feels good right after her break, but an hour later she feels tired and usually has a cup of iced coffee or tea to tide her over until lunch. In the winter, she has hot chocolate at lunch and feels great until about two o'clock, when she takes another break. By then, she's working on a stiff neck and a headache and she takes an aspirin. Her afternoon break is a brownie and another cola. She is behind in her work, so she has to eat it on the run to a staff meeting. The snack and the aspirin usually take her headache away or at least dull it. Since she only had low-fat cottage cheese and a salad for lunch, she decides to splurge on the way home and gets a chocolate milk shake and a double coffee. By the time she gets home, she feels a little jittery and drinks two glasses of wine after her steak dinner so she can get to sleep. She wakes up at 2:00 A.M. and is unable to get back to sleep. Getting up, she takes a sleeping pill that used to work but doesn't seem to anymore. At 4:00 A.M., she is sitting in her kitchen, staring out the window and wondering if she should take another sleeping pill. At 4:30, she opens the freezer and bolts down the rest of a half-gallon of chocolate ice cream. When she goes in for her yearly physical, her physician tells her she has beginning signs of diabetes and her blood pressure is too high. He says her X rays show she has early signs of osteoporosis. She looks at him and says, "How can this happen? I watch what I eat. I'm even on a diet."

SWEETENER STRESS

Eating sugary foods can aggravate tension, increase stress, and add unwanted pounds. They taste good, but the feeling of euphoria—the so-called sugar high—that comes following their ingestion quickly disappears. Meanwhile, your adrenal glands and pancreas are overworked trying to deal with the infusion of sugar. This is stressful and fatiguing. Research shows[1,2,3] that the mood enhancement provided by sugary snacks only lasts for a little while. After one or two hours, fatigue and decreased energy return. When the research subjects increased their intake of sugars, they could only achieve an elevation in mood for a little while.

When this dip in mood occurs, it's common to reach for more sugar. The body, in its wisdom, aims for a balance, and so, following any "high," an extreme low will follow, along with feelings of irritability and fatigue. This leads to *even more* sugar consumption. It may be almost automatic to reach for another sugary food to elevate your mood again. Eat enough sweet foods to get up from the "low" that follows a sugar high and there is no way you are going to lose weight.

This "sugar high–sugar low" reaction is stressful for the emotional state, too. Recent research shows sugar can increase anxiety and depression, two major signs of stress. One study[4] examined the effects of eliminating refined sugar from the diet of twenty moderately to severely depressed volunteers, using the Beck Depression Inventory, a well-respected tool. The researchers concluded that eliminating sugar from the volunteers' diet reduced their symptoms of depression. Three months later, with sugar still eliminated from their diet, the volunteers' symptoms had not returned, showing this was not just a temporary response. There is another major problem with eating sugary delights: insulin resistance. Insulin is one of the hormones the pancreas releases when the blood is full of sugar (blood sugar glucose is elevated). Normally, whenever sugary foods are eaten, more insulin is released to bring blood glucose levels down. Obesity seems to cause an impaired (insulin resistance) response to sugar. Instead of insulin being able to bring blood glucose levels down, the extra sugar is sent to fat depositories on the thighs, buttocks, and belly, where it settles in for long-term storage. Other excess sugar is processed into triglycerides, vicious little fat particles that increase your risk for heart disease.

Eating sweet foods that are low-fat will not help you lose weight. When fat is removed from low-fat foods, it is replaced with sugars. This is even worse in some ways than eating fat. A recent study of twins[5] sheds some interesting light on this and also shows that the tendency toward obesity is not necessarily inherited, as is often assumed. The researchers studied 436 sets of twins, measuring what they ate using a seven-day food diary and a food-frequency questionnaire. They also asked the twins about their activity and whether they smoked or took hormones. There is a widely held belief that eating a lot of dietary fat may lead to overweight, but this study did not bear out that belief. Whether they reported eating high- or low-fat foods, the only twins who were over-weight were the ones who ate a lot of high-sugar (su-crose) foods. It's your insulin resistance and the overconsumption of easily digested sugars in those low-fat cookies or cakes or whatever sugary delights you fa-vor that are the real culprits in the battle of the bulge.

Even if you don't eat sweets, sugar may be added to processed foods and you may not even know it. It is com-mon to add sugar to peas, ravioli, bread, soup, and many other food products. For this reason—and many others—it's important to read labels and know what you're eating. On the nutrition label, make sure none of the sugars to avoid listed here appears as the first four or five ingredi-ents on the list. High-fructose corn syrup is the most ac-tive in triggering the glycation process. Be sure to check labels of everything you eat for these stressors. If you're eating out, you may want to ask the waiter to find out if any of these ingredients are lurking in your food.

To avoid stress, try to avoid these sugars:

- sucrose
- dextrose
- fructose or high-fructose corn syrup
- maltose or malt
- lactose
- honey
- sugarcane
- cane juice

Identifying the Sugars That May Be Stressful for You
Refined sugars are especially bad for you. These are sweeteners that are added to foods to make them taste better, as opposed to *unrefined sugars,* which occur natu-rally in fruits and some vegetables. For example, the sugar in chocolate chip cookies is added, but the sugar in

an orange or banana is a natural sweetener. At least one study has shown[6] that in a comparison of men and women who were overweight and ate the same number of calories as a similar group of lean individuals, those who were overweight ate more refined sugars. So, calories alone are not always the problem.

Foods with added sugar keep the weight on for another reason. These foods usually have so little fiber that they do not move through your intestines quickly. As a result, they may lie in the digestive tract and continue to be absorbed. Overweight individuals may not have the ability to metabolize sugars as easily as lean-bodied people do.

Another stress culprit is eating more refined sugars in combination with high amounts of fat. These troublesome foods taste good and seduce eaters into a cycle of eating more and more of them. The seducers are doughnuts, cookies, cakes, pies, ice cream, candy bars, Danish or sweet rolls, and other baked goods.

How does this seduction occur? It happens because the foods taste good—chalk that up to added sugar—but they are nutritionally unsound, and so they're not satisfying for more than a few hours. This leads to eating more and more sweet foods. Which seducers are your biggest challenge? Take the following Food Seduction Test to find out.

> DIRECTIONS: Place a 1 in front of each sugary seduction food you eat at least once a week, and a 2, 3, 4, etc., for those you eat more than once a week.
>
> ____ doughnuts
>
> ____ cookies
>
> ____ cakes
>
> ____ pies or turnovers

___ ice cream or frozen yogurt

___ pudding

___ candy bars or chocolates

___ sweet rolls, Danish, or other baked goods

___ strawberry shortcake

NOTE: Some of these items also contain trans-fats, which have been shown to contribute to coronary heart disease and accelerated atherosclerosis.

Why You Don't Want Artificial Sweeteners in Your Weight Loss Program

Artificially sweetened foods will not help bypass these problems. They can worsen depression or cause depressive symptoms in some people. In particular, individuals who suffer from mood disorders seem to be more sensitive to artificial sweeteners, like aspartame (NutraSweet and Equal) and experience increased bloating, headaches, and weight gain. Some suspect there may also be a link between synthetic sweeteners like aspartame and saccharine and certain tumors. Reported reactions to aspartame include headaches, mood swings, changes in vision, nausea and diarrhea, sleep disorders, memory loss and confusion, and even convulsions. Finally, aspartame is stressful because it contributes to the formation of formaldehyde in the body.[7,8,9,10]

Avoid aspartame if you have diabetes, are pregnant or prone to confusion or memory loss, or have hypoglycemia. Aspartame also contains methanol—which is known as wood alcohol. Although the Food and Drug Administration states that exposure to methanol through aspartame consumption is not of "sufficient quantity to be of toxicological concern," we just don't know the cumulative effects of high doses of aspartame. Then why are we concerned? Because aspartame is found in so many products that you may be ingesting huge doses and not even know it. Check the following table for the products where aspartame lurks:

SOURCES OF ASPARTAME

Breath mints
Cereals
Chewing gum (sugar-free brands)
Cocoa mix
Coffee beverages
Diet candies
Diet cookies
Diet sodas
Frozen desserts
Gelatin desserts
Instant breakfasts
Juices that are artificially sweetened
Laxatives
Mulitvitamins
Nonprescription drugs
Shake mixes
Tabletop sweeteners
Tea beverages
Instant teas and coffees
Topping mixes
Wine coolers
Yogurts

Some scientific studies suggest that artificial sweeteners can promote hyperactivity and impair the ability to think and learn in children. While other studies show no harmful effects and aspartame is approved by the FDA as safe, that is not always a guarantee, as evidenced by the number of drug recalls, sometimes as much as twelve years after they have been put on the market.

The brain's nourishment depends primarily on glucose. When this sugar enters the brain it is accompanied by natural nutrients found in foods that help balance its effects. Aspartame, which is 200 times sweeter than sugar, is composed of two amino acids, aspartic acid and phenylalanine. Unlike glucose, these chemicals do not provide any nutrition to the brain, nor do they help transport cushioning nutrients; some critics believe they may interfere with neurotransmitters that are responsible for mood, concentration, and learning skills, and that supplying the brain with unnatural substances may cause unnatural behavior.

Artificial sweeteners have also been linked to cancer ever since cyclamate was shown to cause bladder cancer in experimental animals. The FDA banned cyclamate's use in 1968, but subsequent tests have failed to demonstrate that it causes cancer in humans, so it may be reintroduced. Part of the difficulty in making a definitive determination is that results in animal studies can't always be applied to humans. Cyclamate may be a cocarcinogen that only results in malignant growth when it is associated with some other chemical or factor. Other studies that suggest saccharin can also cause bladder cancer led the FDA to propose banning it in 1977, but because of congressional pressure the FDA settled for the following label: "Use of this product may be hazardous to your health. This product contains saccharin, which has been determined to cause cancer in laboratory animals." Aspartame was linked to an increase in brain tumors in a 1996 report, but several subsequent studies strongly dispute this.

With all this controversy, why take a chance when the number of calories saved by substituting a packet or two of aspartame for sugar is really not that great? Despite the many claims, there is no indication that any of the artificial sweeteners currently available or pending approval are truly safe. Natural unrefined and fruit sugars are your best choice.

WHY YOU MAY WANT TO ELIMINATE PROCESSED FOODS

Just as does sugar, consuming too many white, starchy, processed foods can produce insulin resistance and send blood glucose straight to fat depositories. This is because the fiber has been taken out of these white, pasty products. During the refining process, it's all removed, making a doughy, too easily digested starch that can dramatically increase blood glucose levels.

Until recently no one worried about processed foods, but researchers at the Picowe Institute for Medical Research in Manhasset, New York, have shown that high levels of advanced glycation end products (AGEs) from processed foods are absorbed into the blood. These substances accelerate aging and the progress of diseases. When you eat foods that are both sugary and processed, two types of highly stressful substances—sugar and AGEs—are ingested.

CAFFEINE MAY BE STRESSFUL FOR YOU

Caffeine is another substance that can be stressful, yet it is the world's most commonly used mood-altering drug. Nearly 80 percent of the population is addicted to it. It is used to wake up in the morning, despite the fact that the healthy body has its own built-in wake-up clock.

In low doses, caffeine increases feelings of well-being, concentration, and energy levels, but in high doses, it produces jitteriness, restlessness, anxiety, depression, and insomnia—all sources of stress. Not only that, but caffeine also raises blood pressure, contributes to adrenal exhaustion, creates hormonal imbalances, and has even been linked to cancer. Caffeine is listed as a specific poison on page 2687 of *The Merck Manual of Diagnosis and Therapy,* a medical text that has been relied on for 100 years. Symptoms listed as signs of caffeine poisoning include: wakefulness, restlessness, anorexia (no appetite), dehydration, and convulsions. Except for convulsions, these are symptoms that commonly occur when using caffeine.

A study published in the *American Journal of Clinical Nutrition* in 1999[11] showed that homocysteine (a risk factor for heart and blood vessel disease) is positively associated with drinking coffee. It is not unusual to go into a near-panic-attack state from too much caffeine before realizing the symptoms are due to drinking coffee.

At the Department of Public Health at Alicante University[12] scientists have been studying the effect of caffeine on conception. They looked at more than 3,000 women in five countries and charted the consumption of caffeinated beverages versus fecundity (ability to get pregnant). Guess what they found? That's right: the more caffeine a woman took in, the more delayed conception was, and these were women who were healthy in every other way. Another study, at the University of North Carolina at Chapel Hill,[13] also found that caffeine consumption affected fecundability or the monthly probability of conception.

Caffeine also raises blood pressure. A recent study in the *American Journal of Cardiology*[14] examined the effect of caffeine in men with mild high blood pressure, using a sample of twenty-four men with borderline hypertension (140 to 160/90 to 99) and twenty-four healthy men. All the men were tested after twelve hours of caffeine abstinence and an overnight fast. They were tested with a separate caffeine and placebo (sugar pill) about two days apart. Caffeine increased the blood pressure (both systolic and diastolic) and suppressed the heart rate and heart output for all the men, but it was greatest for the men with the already-elevated blood pressure. In fact, they experienced a two to three times greater change in blood pressure compared to the healthy men.

Yet caffeine is so widely consumed in coffee, tea, cocoa, soft drinks (regular and diet), chocolate, and prescription and over-the-counter drugs that it is hard not to ingest high levels of the substance. When trying to lose weight, try not to add more stress in the form of caffeine. Unlike most other drugs, caffeine is unregulated and its presence in food and beverages is often hidden. Anyone who has tried to quit using this drug knows it's addictive. Quitting cold turkey can result in headaches, irritability, and fatigue. As with any addictive drug, there is a withdrawal period. Fortunately, with caffeine it only lasts a day or so. It's also possible to be caffeine-dependent and not even realize it. A self-test question for caffeine dependency is: "Can I get up and function without at least one cup of coffee in the morning?" If the answer is no, caffeine dependency or even addiction exists. The dependency or addiction need not be to coffee; chocolate and colas also qualify. They all siphon off energy, increase stress, exert a letdown reaction (so more is needed in an hour or so), and decrease your overall mental activity.

Although there is controversy about coffee and some studies show no negative effects from drinking a cup or two a day, even a little caffeine can be problematic for some people. It's important to identify your healthy balance to reduce unneeded stress.

How Caffeine Could Harm Your Nutrient Balance

Since caffeine is a diuretic, it leaches B vitamins out of your body. This is a problem because B vitamins promote good digestion and metabolism, help with tissue repair and formation, dissolve cholesterol, aid in proper mental functioning, enhance mood, lower homocysteine levels (see p. 47), assist in the production of body energy, and, most important for you, help with the metabolism of fats and carbohydrates.

If you do ingest caffeine, consider eating foods high in B vitamins or taking a B-vitamin supplement to protect yourself from heart disease and other conditions related to B-vitamin deficiency.[15] B vitamins are not the only nutrients leeched out of your body when you use caffeine. Calcium and magnesium also go out in your urine.[16]

Calcium is a very important mineral that keeps bones and teeth strong. It also is important in warding off osteoporosis. Avoid taking the chance of having unnecessary broken bones and the crippling bowed-over back that comes with osteoporosis. Calcium also does much more, and you really need it. This mineral is important in keeping your heart beating regularly, lowering cholesterol levels, and helping prevent heart disease and in the transmission of nerve impulses. It also prevents muscle cramps, is essential in blood clotting, and may help prevent cancer. Calcium, along with vitamin D, may have an important role in the prevention of colorectal cancer.[17] It helps break down fats for metabolism and utilization by the body. This mineral also keeps your cells and skin healthy, helps your muscles move correctly, and protects against eclampsia, the number-one cause of maternal death. Without enough calcium, symptoms such as aching joints, brittle nails, eczema, elevated cholesterol, heart palpitations, high blood pressure, muscle cramps, numbness in the arms and/or legs, a pasty complexion, rheumatoid arthritis, rickets, tooth decay, insomnia, and nervousness occur.

Calcium may also protect you from the stress of cancer. A recent report from the Division of Cancer Prevention and Control of the National Cancer Institute[18] stated that dietary (epidemiological) studies suggest that calcium can help prevent certain cancers. Trials using calcium, vitamin E, and vitamin D are now under way, aimed at lung and colorectal cancer. Another study,[19] by J. A. Baron and colleagues, found that calcium protects against cancer of the colon and rectum, while pilot studies in Europe have cleared the way for large-scale trials of calcium, vitamins A, C, and E, and the B-vitamin folic acid to reduce cancer.

Magnesium is another mineral that is important to a calm and healthy life. As this mineral is necessary for calcium uptake and magnesium losses can occur due to caffeine, ingesting caffeine interferes with healthy calcium levels in two ways! One study of normal adult women found that just one cup of a beverage that contains six milligrams of caffeine increased total urine output of water, magnesium, sodium, chloride, potassium, and creatine for two hours following ingestion.[20]

A deficiency of magnesium interferes with the ability

to transmit nerve and muscle impulses and leads to irritability and nervousness. Magnesium is also the essential mineral that protects arterial linings from stress caused by sudden blood pressure changes. Other studies found that magnesium reduced heart arrhythmias as well as some drug treatments[21] and without the side effects and that magnesium intake was lower in patients with heart arrhythmias than in those without irregular heartbeats.[22]

Infrequently, dietary imbalances, such as high intakes of fat and/or calcium, can intensify magnesium deficiency. This can happen especially under conditions of stress. Magnesium can protect the body from stress in other ways. Studies show that magnesium is one of the key protectors against diabetes[23,24] and that preterm delivery in women can be stopped by using one form of magnesium.[25] This mineral may even be linked to the HDL (good form of) cholesterol.[26] A large body of evidence also suggests that magnesium may keep blood pressure low[27,28] and may even protect you against kidney stones.[29] So, hold onto your magnesium stores and cut back on caffeine.

As you can see, consuming caffeine can actually prevent your body from being healthy and from losing the weight you want to lose. Be sure you're not taking in stressful caffeine and hidden (and not so hidden) sources by consulting the list that follows.

IS CAFFEINE STRESSING YOU OUT?

DIRECTIONS: Check off all the sources of caffeine that may be stressing you. Depending on your circumstances, even one may be too many, but if you're regularly using two or more, we suggest you switch to noncaffeinated substitutes. (See the next chapter for what to use instead.) Monitor your daily caffeine intake by checking off the ones you ingest and calcualting the amount of caffeine you are consuming.

NUMBER OF MG. OF DAILY CAFFEINE

Coffee, 5-ounce cup

____ drip coffee: number of cups x 130 mg. = mg.

____ espresso, single shot (Starbucks) = 80 mg.

____ instant coffee = 65 mg.

____ decaffeinated, brewed = 3 mg.

____ decaffeinated, instant = 2 mg.

Tea, 5-ounce cup

____ 1-minute brewed hot tea: number of cups x 20 mg. = mg.

____ 3-minute brewed hot tea: number of cups x 35 mg. = mg.

____ 12 ounces iced tea: number of glasses x 70 mg. = mg.

Drugs

____ over-the-counter drugs that contain caffeine (check the label for ingredients in other drugs)

____ No-Doz = 100 mg.

____ Vivarin = 200 mg.

____ Anacin (pain relief) = 32 mg.

____ Excedrin (pain relief) = 65 mg.

____ Midol (menstrual pain) = 32 mg.

____ Vanquish (pain relief) = 33 mg.

____ Aqua Ban Plus (diuretic) = 200 mg.

____ prescription drugs that contain caffeine (ask your pharmacist about other drugs)

____ Cafergot (for migraine headache) = 100 mg.

____ Florinal (for tension headache) = 40 mg.

____ Soma Compound (for pain/muscle relaxant) = 32 mg.

____ Darvon Compound (for pain) = 32 mg.

Chocolate (in any form from candy to cocoa—a double whammy: sugar and caffeine!)

____ cocoa, 5-ounce cup = 4 mg.

____ chocolate milk, 8 ounces = 5 mg.

____ milk chocolate, 1 ounce = 6 mg.

____ dark chocolate, semisweet, 1 ounce = 20 mg.

____ baker's chocolate, 1 ounce = 26 mg.

____ chocolate-flavored syrup, 1 ounce = 4 mg.

Soft drinks, 12-ounce serving

____ Canada Dry Diet Cola = 1 mg.

____ Canada Dry Jamaica Cola = 30 mg.

____ Diet-Rite = 36 mg.

____ RC Cola = 36 mg.

____ Pepsi Light = 36 mg.

____ Diet Pepsi = 36 mg.

____ Aspen = 36 mg.

____ Pepsi-Cola = 38 mg.

____ Diet Dr Pepper = 40 mg.

____ Shasta Cola or Cherry Cola = 44 mg.

____ Diet Coke = 46 mg.

____ Coca-Cola = 46 mg.

____ Mello Yello = 53 mg.

____ Mountain Dew = 54 mg.

____ Diet Mr. PiBB = 59 mg.

NOW ADD UP YOUR TOTAL MGS. OF DAILY CAFFEINE: ____

Think about reducing or eliminating caffeine from your meal plan.

(SOURCES: National Soft Drink Association; *FDA Consumer*, 1984)

HOW GLUTEN MAY BE STRESSING YOU

Foods that contain gluten may be stressful for your body. For individuals sensitive to this substance, every time a gluten-containing food is eaten, a portion of the lining of the small intestine is damaged. This creates a great deal of stress in the intestine and makes it nearly impossible to absorb vital stress-reducing nutrients, including vitamins A, D, and K, iron, potassium, vitamin B_{12}, and calcium. This can result in severe nutrient deficiencies.

Research also indicates that environmental factors, such as gluten intolerance, contribute to diabetes. In one study[30] researchers found a substantially lower diabetes incidence in mice on a gluten-free diet compared to mice on a standard diet. These findings from animal studies may not have a direct correlation to humans, but they do provide more evidence for the effect of gluten on insulin function and particularly diabetes.

Symptoms of gluten intolerance include abdominal cramping, gas, bloating, chronic diarrhea or constipation (sometimes both), fatigue, depression, and bone or joint pain after eating any foods with the following grains in them: wheat, rye, oats, barley, triticale, kamut, or spelt. For the gluten-intolerant, gluten may be increasing these uncomfortable and unhealthy symptoms and interfering with normal digestion that can help maintain a healthy weight. If you have these symptoms consider staying away from gluten. It is found in breads, cakes, pies, cereals, and canned goods. Be sure to read labels of everything you eat. If you're eating in a restaurant, think about just staying away from these items.

OXIDIZED TRANS-FATS AND MARGARINE STRESS

The American diet is particularly high in oxidized fats, most of which are in the form of trans-fats or trans-fatty acids. These products were developed by food-processing companies through a production process called hydrogenation, which transforms vegetable oils into more solid substances that resist spoiling and behave more like butter or lard during baking and frying. The resultant trans-fat compounds are quite different in chemical composition from the fatty acids naturally present in food and have far more serious effects. They decrease HDL (good cholesterol), increase LDL (bad cholesterol), and can cause diabetes by interfering with insulin receptors, so the pancreas has to constantly manufacture more insulin and eventually becomes exhausted. Trans-fat chemicals can also alter the composition, size, and number of your fat cells, promoting weight gain. They can contribute to cancer by accelerating the malignant changes started by various carcinogens.

Trans-fats are found in almost all commercially made doughnuts, crackers, cookies, pastries, fried foods, potato and corn chips, baked goods, frosting, candy products, and margarine. For most Americans, fried foods are the biggest source of trans-fats. A medium order of fast-food French fries contains four to five times as much trans-fat as one teaspoon of stick margarine. One survey of 85,000 nurses[31] confirmed that those who consumed more of these oxidized trans-fat foods, and especially margarine, had higher rates of both heart disease and cancer.

Margarine was originally touted as a substitute that would taste the same as butter but reduce the risk for heart attacks and other atherosclerotic complications. Now it appears that margine may be just as harmful as butter or even more so. Hard stick margarines have undergone more hydrogenation and contain twice as many trans-fats as softer products that come in tubs. Margarines that can be sprayed or squeezed on foods or cooking utensils may be the best option, but you're better off using olive oil.

MEAT AND ANIMAL PRODUCT STRESS

Eating too many meat and animal products (eggs, cheese, milk) can also stress the kidneys and liver and leaves less room for the fruits, vegetables, and grains. This stress is exacerbated when you consume meat from animals who have received antibiotics, hormones, and other drugs that may be passed on to you. If you must eat meat or poultry, look into eating organically grown animals that do not contain drugs.

A more vegetarianlike eating plan is associated not only with a lower weight but also with less heart disease, diabetes, and other chronic illness.[32,33,34,35] For these reasons alone, consider eating more vegetables, fruits, and grains and fewer animal products.

There is a longer term, perhaps more important, reason to limit intake of meat and animal products. Almost three decades ago, Dr. Kilmer McCully proposed that the culprit in coronary heart disease was not cholesterol but a chemical called homocysteine. Homocysteine is derived from methionine, an essential amino acid found in meats and animal products. McCulley proposed that eating too much of these foods could be harmful not because they contained too much cholesterol but because they contained high levels of methionine. Under normal circumstances, certain B-complex vitamins metabolize methionine and homocysteine into compounds that are useful and safe. Meats and dairy products are low in these B vitamins, which are found mainly in fresh fruits and vegetables, but if you don't eat enough fruits and vegetables and eat a diet too high in meat and animal products, you will suffer the stress of elevated homocysteine that can eventually cause physical damage to your heart.

CHEMICAL ADDITIVES, DYES, PESTICIDES, AND PRESERVATIVES

Many Americans eat processed meat and dairy products, including sandwich meats, bacon, processed cheese foods, hot dogs, and other canned, boxed, and preserved (usually with nitrites and/or nitrates) meats. Many of these processed foods contain chemical additives, dyes, and preservatives, which may be stressing your body. When these foods are processed, most of the important B vitamins that help you metabolize homocysteine, the heart-damaging substance described earlier, are destroyed. To protect your heart, avoid processed foods.

Unless organically grown, vegetables, fruits, and grains are treated with pesticides. Although many of the more toxic pesticides have been banned in the United States, they can be used in other countries and the tainted produce can then be shipped back here for sale. (More recently, these foods are grown using genetic engineering processes, although there have been no long-term studies to investigate the long-term effects of these approaches—another reason to use organically grown foods.)

Pesticides work by blocking the action of specific enzymes that control life processes in plants, insects, and fungi. While the pesticide levels in food may be low and seem to be harmless, the chemicals can accumulate in body fat. Over time, they can inflame tissues and damage the genetic code in cells. While the liver usually enhances health by filtering out toxins, it can only filter out toxins that are water-soluble, not fat-soluble. Pesticides are fat-soluble. As the myelin sheath that protects the brain is made of fat, toxins from pesticides may be stored there. This can lead to memory loss through depressing or blocking the flow of acetyl-choline, the main message carrier in memory cells.

Some food flavor enhancers can also be stressful. The chief flavor enhancer that excites the brain in a stressful way (excitotoxin) is MSG, or monosodium glutamate. Manufacturers of processed foods may mislead consumers and disguise this excitotoxin. See the following table for a listing of some commonly used names for MSG or products that often contain this substance.

The best way to avoid additives, dyes, pesticides, and preservatives is to use organically grown foods. Grow your own foods whenever you can and check with your local health food stores and grocery stores for sources of organically grown produce. Caring for a vegetable garden or at least an herb garden is also a good way to decrease stress. All you need is a windowsill or a sunny area and a tiny pot or two. Check with your local nursery for tips.

FOOD FLAVOR ENHANCERS THAT MAY CONTAIN MSG: STEER CLEAR!

Look on the label of any processed foods for the following ingredients and try to avoid them, as they may contain MSG:

Hydrolyzed anything (oat flour, plant protein, or vegetable protein)
Plant protein extract
Textured protein
Yeast extract
Bouillon
Broth
Malt extract, malt flavoring, natural beef or chicken flavoring
Seasoning spices
Carrageenan
Enzymes
Soy or whey protein concentrate or isolate

ALLERGIES OR FOOD SENSITIVITIES MAY BE STRESSING YOU AND KEEPING YOU OVERWEIGHT

Researchers at the Health and Medical Research Foundation in San Antonio[36] recruited 100 overweight individuals who had at least two other food-allergy symptoms, such as intestinal disturbances and migraines. They weighed and measured each person for fat-to-lean ratio and asked each of them to complete a Disease Symptom inventory and take a blood test that identified food sensitivities. Half the group were then given the blood test results and asked to eliminate the offending foods from their diets. After thirty days, the group who had avoided allergens had lost an average of nearly three pounds of fat and had gained almost one pound of lean muscle. They also reported a significant reduction in disease symptoms, while the control group, the other fifty people, who had chosen their own diet, gained an average of one pound of fat, lost almost one pound of lean muscle, and reported minimal improvement in their disease symptoms.

One clue that you might have a food allergy is an irritating cough or tickle in your throat. To find out if the symptom is an allergic reaction, stop eating the food and see if the symptom subsides. Then reintroduce the food and see if the symptom reappears. Identify any food allergens and avoid them if you want to lose weight and keep it off!

TAKING ACTION TO REDUCE FOOD STRESS
Be sure to set a goal or two for eliminating stressful foods. Use the following form or devise one of your own:

____ I will stop using aspartame (NutraSweet) or eating any foods or drinking any drinks that contain it as of tomorrow.

____ I will stop using caffeine by the end of this week.

____ After today, I won't buy candy bars anymore and will ask my family not to bring them in the house or car.

____ I'm going to eliminate white bread and pasta from my diet and use whole-grain products instead.

____ I will eat one less meat serving a day starting Sunday.

____ I will not eat fried foods or use margarine after today.

____ I will start using organically grown foods for at least one meal a day by next week.

REFERENCES

1. Christensen, L. 1991. The role of caffeine and sugar in depression. *Nutrition Report* 9(3):17–24.
2. Christensen, L. 1993. Effects of eating behavior on mood: A review of the literature. *International Journal of Eating Disorders* 14:171–83.
3. Christensen, L., and C. Redig. 1993. Effect of meal composition on mood. *Behavioral Neuroscience* 107:346–53.
4. Christensen, L., and R. Burrows. 1990. Dietary treatment of depression. *Behavior Therapy* 21.
5. Samaras, K., P. J. Kellyu, M. N. Chiano, N. Arden, T. D. Spector, and L. V. Campbell. 1998. Genes versus environment: The relationship between dietary fat and total and central abdominal fat. *Diabetes Care* 21(12): 2069–76.
6. Miller, W. C., M. G. Niederpruem, J. P. Wallace, A. K. Lindeman. 1994. Dietary fat, sugar and fiber predict body fat content. *Journal of the American Dietary Association* 94(6): 612–15.
7. Van den Eeden, S. K., T. D. Koepsell, W. T. Longstreth, G. van Belle, J. R. Daling, and B. McKnight. 1994. Aspartame ingestion and headaches: A randomized crossover trial. *Neurology* 44(10): 1787–93.
8. Walton, R. G., R. Hudak, and R. J. Green-Waite. 1993. Adverse reactions to aspartame double-blind challenge in patients from a vulnerable population. *Biological Psychiatry* 34(1–2): 13–17.
9. Olney, J. W., N. B. Farber, E. Spitznagel, and L. N. Robins. 1996. Increasing brain tumor rates: Is there a link to aspartame? *Journal of Neuropathology and Experimental Neurology* 55(11): 1115–23.
10. Trocho, C., R. Pardo, I. Rafecas, J. Virgili, X. Remesar, J. A. Fernandex-Lopez, and M. Alemany. 1998. Formaldehyde derived from dietary aspartame binds to tissue components in vivo. *Life Science* 63(5): 337–39.
11. El-Khairy, L., P. M. Ueland, O. Nygard, H. Refsum, and S. E. Vollset. 1999. Lifestyle and cardiovascular disease risk factors as determinants of total cysteine in plasma: The Hordaland Homocysteine Study. *American Journal of Clinical Nutrition* 70(6): 1016–24.
12. Bolumar, F., J. Olsen, M. Rebagliato, and L. Bisanti. 1997.

Caffeine intake and delayed conception: A European multi-center study on infertility and subfecundity. *American Journal of Epidemiology* 145(4): 324–34.

13. Curtis, K. M., D. A. Savitz, and T. E. Arbuckle. 1997. Effects of cigarette smoking, caffeine consumption and alcohol intake on fecundability. *American Journal of Epidemiology* 146(1): 32–41.

14. Pincomb, A., W. R. Lovallo, B. S. McKey, B. Hee Sung, R. B. Passey, S. A. Everson, and M. F. Wilson. 1996. Acute blood pressure elevations with caffeine in men with borderline systemic hypertension. *American Journal of Cardiology* 77: 270–74.

15. Chait, A., M. R. Malinow, D. C. Morris, et al. 1999. Increased dietary micronutrients decrease serum homocysteine concentrations in patients at high risk of cardiovascular disease. *American Journal of Clinical Nutrition* 70: 881–87.

16. Kynast-Gales, S. A., and L. K. Massey. 1994. Effect of caffeine on circadian excretion of urinary calcium and magnesium. *Journal of the American College of Nutrition* 13(5): 467–72.

17. Lipkin, M. 1999. Preclinical and early human studies of calcium and cancer prevention. *Annals of the New York Academy of Sciences* 889: 120–27.

18. Greenwald, P., and S. S. McDonald. 1997. Cancer prevention: The roles of diet and chemoprevention. *Cancer Control* 4(2): 118–27.

19. Baron, J. A., M. Beach, J. S. Mandel, R. U. van Stolk, R. Haile, R. Rothstein, R. W. Summers, D. C. Snover, G. J. Beck, L. Francis, J. H. Bond, E. R. Greenberg. 1999. Calcium supplements and colorectal adenomas: Prevention Study Group. *Annals of the New York Academy of Science* 889: 138–45.

20. Bergman, E. A., L. K. Massey, K. J. Wise, and D. J. Sherrard 1990. Effects of dietary caffeine on renal handling of normal women. *Life Science* 47(6): 557–64.

21. Brodsky, M. A., et al. 1994. Magnesium therapy in new-onset atrial fibrillation. *American Journal of Cardiology* 73: 1227–29.

22. Singh, P. H., and G. E. Fraser. 1998. Dietary risk factors for

colon cancer in a low-risk population. *American Journal of Epidemiology* 148(8): 761–74.

23. Meyer, K. A., L. H. Kushi, D. R. Jacobs, J. Slavin, and P. Sellers. 2000. Carbohydrates, dietary fiber and incident type 2 diabetes in older women. *American Journal of Clinical Nutrition* 71(4): 921–30.

24. Kao, W. H., A. R. Folsom, F. J. Nieto, J. P. Mo, and R. L. Watson. 1999. Serum and dietary magnesium and the risk for type 2 diabetes mellitus: The atherosclerosis risk in communities. *Archives of Internal Medicine* 159(18): 2151–59.

25. Haghighi, L. 1999. Prevention of preterm delivery: Nifedipine or magnesium sulfate. *International Journal of Gynaecology and Obstetrics* 66(3): 297–98.

26. Nozue, T., N. Ide, H. Okabe, K. Narui, and A. Kobayashi. 1999. Correlation of serum HDL-cholesterol and LCA T in the fraction of ionized magnesium in children. *Magnesium Research* 12(4): 297–301.

27. Rude, R. K., M. E. Kirchen, H. E. Gruber, M. H. Meyer, and D. L. Luck. 1999. Magnesium deficiency–induced osteoporosis in the uncoupling of bone formation and bone resorption. *Magnesium Research* 12(4): 257–67.

28. Tucker, K. L., M. T. Hannan, H. Chen, L. A. Cupples, and R. Wilson. 1999. Potassium, magnesium and fruit and vegetable intake associated with greater bone mineral density in elderly men and women. *American Journal of Clinical Nutrition* 69(4): 727–36.

29. Celotti, F., and A. Bignamini. 1999. Dietary calcium and mineral/vitamin supplementation. *Journal of Internal Medicine Research* 27(1): 1–14.

30. Funda, D. P., A. Kaas, T. Bock, H. Tlaskalova-Hogenova, and K. Bushard. 1999. Gluten-free diets prevent diabetes in NOD mice. *Diabetes Metabolism Research Review* 15(5): 323–27.

31. Rosch, P. 1999. Oxidized trans-fats and margarines. *Health and Stress* 8: 4–5.

32. Key, T. J., G. E. Fraser, M. Thorogood, P. N. Appleby, R. Beral, M. L. Burr, J. Chang-Claude, R. Frentzel-Beyme, T. Kuzma, and K. McPherson. 1998. Mortality in vegetarians and non-vegetarians: An analysis of 8,300 deaths among

76,000 men and women in prospective studies. *Public Health Nutrition* 1(1): 33–41.

33. Key, T. J., G. E. Fraser, M. Thorogood, P. N. Appleby, R. Beral, M. L. Burr, J. Chang-Claude, R. Frentzel-Beyme, T. Kuzma, and K. McPherson. 1999. Mortality in vegetarians and nonvegetarians: Derived from a collaborative analysis of 5 prospective studies. *American Journal of Clinical Nutrition* 70(3 Supplement): 516S–524S.

34. Fraser, G. E. 1999. Diet as primordial prevention in Seventh-Day Adventists. *Preventive Medicine* 29(6, pt. 2): S18–S22.

35. Fraser, G. E. 1999. Associations between diet and cancer, ischemic heart disease and all-cause mortality in non-Hispanic white Caucasian Seventh-Day Adventists. *American Journal of Clinical Nutrition* 70(3 Supplement): 532S–538S.

36. Unpublished study at the Health and Medical Research Foundation, San Antonio, Texas.

CHAPTER 4

Step 3: Start Filling Up on Food in a Stress-Less Way to Lose Weight

A faulty diet can be both a source of stress for your body and a result of the emotional stress that can lead to poor eating habits. Some dietary tips that are important for a stress-less lifestyle are:

1. Eat a variety of foods, making sure you listen to your body's "fullness" signals so that you don't overeat.
2. Be sure to include plenty of vegetables, fruits, and whole grains in your diet.
3. Limit your intake of refined sugar, salt, and alcohol.
4. Avoid foods high in sodium, saturated fat, and cholesterol.
5. Drink at least eight glasses of water a day.
6. Make sure you have an adequate intake of essential nutrients and vitamins.

DRINK ENOUGH WATER TO REDUCE STRESS AND HELP YOU DIGEST

During your normal daily activities your body loses about ten cups of water. When you are under stress, during exercise or because of heat, even more water is needed. (Remember that coffee and cola drinks are not good substitutes because they contain caffeine, which flushes even more water out of the system.)

There is another reason to drink water. All chemical reactions that help transform food into energy in the body require water. The brain is about 75 percent water by weight and is the first part of the body to be affected by too little water (dehydration). Although you may not notice, this dehydration can affect mental and physical performance or lead to headaches or fatigue.

Sip water throughout the day. Keep a glass and a pitcher of water handy. You might also want to use lemon slices or fresh berries to enhance the taste.

EAT FIVE OR SIX SMALL MEALS A DAY TO REDUCE CRAVINGS

If you suffer from low blood sugar due to a triggering of insulin production after eating, you may experience sugar craving, depression, weakness, fatigue, jitteriness, palpitations, or headache. Eating five or six small meals that are high in protein and low in carbohydrates at spaced intervals can often produce relief.

EAT EARLIER IN THE DAY FOR LESS STRESS AND MORE WEIGHT LOSS

A study that appeared in the April 2000 issue of *Medicine and Science in Sports and Exercise*[1] backs this up. It showed that eating light all day but having a large evening meal made the participants store more fat. Even though they reduced their daily calories and exercised vigorously, there was no weight loss, and their fat deposits increased—some of the participants actually gained weight. Even more astonishing, these were young female gymnasts with an average age of fifteen and runners with an average age of twenty-seven. They wrote down on an hourly basis exactly what they ate and how much they exercised. The information was fed into a computer that gave an hour-by-hour breakdown of whether they stored more calories than they burned or were burning more calories than they stored. Body fat was also measured. Athletes who burned more calories than they took in tended to have the most body fat, and those who stayed closest to caloric balance throughout the day tended to be leaner. Those who ate a big meal at the end of the day stored it as fat.

There is no law that states that you should eat three meals a day, with the largest one in the evening. This schedule may be sending the wrong signals to your body. In fact, reversing the order of the amount of food eaten can reduce the stress you may be placing yourself in by eating a large meal at night and then not using the calories.

Try eating your largest meal in the morning for a few weeks and see how you feel, what you weigh, how well you sleep, and how well you seem to be metabolizing your food (bowel movements, gas, and intestinal soreness are some clues). Next, eat your biggest meal at lunchtime and again note how you feel, how well you sleep, and how you digest your food. Now, switch to having your biggest meal at night for a few weeks. What differences do you notice?

You'll probably find that eating the most food earlier in the day will lead to losing weight and feeling better. If you eat a big meal late in the day, when you are far less active, the food will just sit in your digestive system. Rather than being metabolized into energy, it will turn into fat. It may even make it difficult for you to sleep. Remember that if you want to lose weight, eat your main meal early in the day—the earlier the better.

LET COOKING AND FOOD SHOPPING REDUCE YOUR STRESS

Cooking can be therapeutic and stress-reducing, if you do it when you're not starving and if you allow enough time to enjoy the process. If you are really hungry when you start to cook, snack on apple slices or a handful of raw sunflower seeds. Cooking is really a labor of love and deserves your full attention. Throw a pinch of dulse or a bit of nutritional yeast into your next soup or tomato sauce. Make it fun. Don't worry about following a recipe exactly; it's only a guideline, not set in stone.

Cooking is something you give yourself, so be creative and enjoy! Put on an apron that suits you and some relaxing music and delight in the smells as your meal begins to cook. Enjoy the sight of a perfect pepper or a well-formed egg or green pea. Enjoy the feel and sound as you slice into a yellow squash or mince onions or parsley. Try a new ingredient in a recipe. Try layering slices of papaya on the next piece of fish you broil, or stuff a green pepper with crab meat and bake it next to your potatoes. Pay attention to the sights, sounds, and smells as you cook and look forward to how good your meal is going to taste when it is ready to eat.

Shopping for a meal for yourself can also be a stress-reducing and pleasing journey if you're creative. Pride yourself on finding an out-of-the way ethnic grocery shop or a local produce stand with bins of fragrant vegetables. Try to buy organically grown foods that have not been grown with pesticides or antibiotics (two stressors). If organic foods aren't available, ask your local food store to supply them or purchase in-season fruits and vegetables from local farmers or produce stands.

Any extra substances, like pesticides sprayed on your fruits and vegetables or antibiotics ingested by the animals you eat, put additional stress on you because your kidneys and liver must work harder to eliminate them from your body. Unnecessary antibiotics are a particular hazard for two reasons. First, they disrupt the balance of probiotic bacteria in your digestive tract. (These are the beneficial bacteria found mainly in yogurt and fermented foods that promote health and help you digest your food.)

Unfortunately, antibiotics don't know the difference between healthy digestive bacteria and bacteria that can cause illness. All of them are obliterated. A recent overview of the use of antibiotics found that the tremendous therapeutic advantage afforded by antibiotics is being threatened by the emergence of increasingly resistant strains of microbes. This is due to the misuse and overuse of antibiotics, including feeding it to animals to reduce their infections when they are raised in crowded conditions.[2,3] Using organic foods will help you avoid the stress of added antibiotics.

If your life is fast-paced, you may only be able to cook with relish on weekends, but do give yourself permission to enjoy the pleasures of cooking and eating your own productions at least once or twice a week. You may also want to rethink why your life is so fast-paced and take steps to slow down. See chapters 5–8 for ideas on how to do that.

EAT MORE ANTIOXIDANT FRUITS, VEGETABLES, AND NUTS FOR LESS STRESS

Another way to reduce physical stress and lose weight, too, is to fill up on antioxidant fruits and vegetables. These foods protect the body from internal and external wear and tear that accelerates the body's production of those tissue-damaging molecules called free radicals. Free radical activity is increased by smoking and by stress and by the process of aging. If this activity is not held in check by natural antioxidants, free radical damage can lead to atherosclerosis, cancer, cataracts, gray hair, and wrinkled skin and other lesions. Antioxidants in some foods are like knights on white horses, attaching themselves to free radicals, rendering them harmless. Examine the following list of vegetables and fruits high in vitamins C and E and beta-carotene, three of the most potent antioxidants, and try to add these foods to your diet:

FOODS HIGH IN VITAMINS C AND E AND BETA-CAROTENE

HIGH-VITAMIN-C FOODS	HIGH-VITAMIN-E FOODS	HIGH-BETA-CAROTENE FOODS
Oranges	Almonds	Carrots
Grapefruits	Wheat germ	Broccoli
Tangerines	Olive oil	Sweet potatoes
Green peppers	Nutritional yeast	Apricots
Honeydew melons	Peanuts	Cantaloupes
Cooked broccoli	Outer leaf of cabbage	Squash
Cantaloupes	Raw spinach	
Papaya	Whole-grain rice	
Brussels sprouts	Asparagus	
Cooked cauliflower	Cornmeal	
Parsley	Eggs	
Onions	Sweet potatoes	
Tomatoes	Leafy portions of broccoli or cauliflower	
Kale		
Raspberries		
Strawberries		

Nuts provide free radical protection through their monounsaturated fats and flavonoids, the antioxidants that fight aging and stress. Nuts also furnish other stress-reducing substances: fiber that fights constipation; calcium and potassium that help steady your blood pressure; and zinc, iron, and magnesium that fight fatigue. Eating five ounces or more of nuts a week is associated with a reduced risk of coronary heart disease in women.[4] Nuts that have demonstrated their worth in research studies for reducing the risk of heart disease include almonds, pecans, macadamias, hazelnuts, pistachios, and walnuts,[5,6,7,8] so you might want to start with those.

Certain foods can help you digest your food, thereby reducing digestive stress, especially if you are an older adult whose digestive enzymes aren't what they used to be. (Unfortunately, digestive enzymes weaken with age.) Try eating a small portion of fresh pineapple or papaya at the end of your meal. They have enzymes (bromelain) that help digest your food by breaking down protein. They also protect against any unfriendly bacteria that may be lurking in your digestive system. If the fresh fruits are unavailable, try canned pineapple in its own juice. Although it won't have as much bromelain in it, the canned version is an alternative. (Remember, you don't want to burden your system with extra processed sugars, so buy the fruit in its own juice.) You can also chew on digestive enzymes. Find them at health food stores.

REDUCE STRESS AND EAT LESS WITH HIGH-SATISFACTION COMPLEX CARBOHYDRATES

Carbohydrates make you feel better. But don't reach for that simple-carbohydrate-laden sugary delight that will only lead to eating too much and the inevitable down that follows when your blood sugar dips again. Instead, grab an apple or a couple of cups of hot-air-popped popcorn. (Keep popcorn already popped in a jar on your counter and a bowl of fruit there, too, so you won't be tempted in a moment of weakness to head for the refrigerator.) You'll feel better quickly because the complex carbohydrates in the apple or popcorn will lift your mood. See the following list of foods that satisfy but also can lead to weight loss. The other good thing about complex carbohydrates is that you won't end up berating yourself for sneaking "forbidden" food. So, have that handful of grapes or slice of whole-wheat bread or a bowl of bran cereal and congratulate yourself because you've eaten something nourishing, not depleting. It could do wonders for the old self-esteem.

Not long ago, if you were trying to lose weight, you may have avoided bread, potatoes, and pasta because you believed these "starchy" foods went right to the hips, but

HIGH-SATISFACTION FOODS

The following foods are ranked in order of the "fullness" factor. They keep you feeling full and satisfied, so you won't reach for sugary sweets or other non-nutritious foods:

Potatoes	Popcorn
Fish	Bran cereal
Oatmeal	Eggs
Oranges	Cheese
Apples	White rice
Whole-wheat pasta	Lentils
Baked beans	Brown rice
Grapes	Rice crackers
Whole-grain bread	

research has proven differently. You can lose more weight and keep it off if you eat foods high in complex carbohydrates, including rice, beans, starchy vegetables, and pasta, because they have a lower "energy density"; that is, they weigh more than high-fat foods but contain fewer calories, says Barbara Rolls, Ph.D., professor of nutrition at Pennsylvania State University in University Park.[9] The lower a food's energy density, the more likely it will fill you up.

Suppose you decided to eat 1,600 calories a day. To get that many calories from high-carbohydrate foods, you would have to eat seventeen whole-wheat pancakes, eleven baked potatoes, eight cups of spaghetti, or eight toasted cinnamon-raisin bagels. Now, let's see what you can eat for 1,600 calories of high-fat foods. The answer is: three fast-food fish sandwiches with cheese and tartar sauce.

When you eat high-carbohydrate foods, you feel satisfied more quickly and don't eat so much. What's more, research has shown that most people prefer following a high-carbohydrate, low-fat diet. That makes sense, because those foods are more filling. If you want to lose weight, select high-fiber foods as your cabohydrate choices. That way, you'll avoid food cravings and hunger pangs and you'll get the nutrients you need to avoid dips in your blood sugar that make you feel depressed and want to reach for more sugary foods.

Snacking on healthy, complex-carbohydrate foods before lunch or dinner will help you to be less apt to overeat at mealtime, but stay away from those fat-free and high-fat snacks (except maybe once a week as a special treat for being such a good person), because you can't depend on them to keep you feeling full and satisfied. Instead, select your snacks from foods that are naturally low in fat and naturally high in fiber: fruits, vegetables, and whole grains.

EAT FOODS HIGH IN FIBER TO REDUCE STRESS TO YOUR DIGESTIVE SYSTEM AND LOSE WEIGHT

Moderate consumption of fiber can help you lose weight and can enhance the workings of your digestive system and help maintain a healthy colon. Remember, cancer of the colon is associated with a low-fiber diet!

One reason fiber can help you lose weight is it gives you a feeling of fullness and makes it easier to limit your intake of food. Another reason is that eating a fibrous food, such as an apple, physically takes longer than digesting a nonfibrous food, such as apple juice. Fibrous foods are also more satisfying. Although apple juice may taste sweet and delicious, it makes you want more. After eating an apple, you will feel full and satisfied. If you don't, eat another. It's no big deal calorie-wise.

If you eat more digestible fibers from breakfast cereals, fruits, vegetables, beans, whole-grain breads, nuts, and seeds, not only will it help you regulate sugar in your body—key to feeling balanced and satisfied—but it also will lower the risk of heart disease and cholesterol. Even indigestible fiber can produce a feeling of fullness useful in weight loss. Psyllium husk powder, an indigestible fiber available at health food stores, can also reduce constipation, abdominal discomfort, and heartburn.[10]

REDUCE CRAVINGS AND SLEEP BETTER WITH TRYPTOPHAN

If you're a woman, you may experience carbohydrate craving and depression before your menstrual period. If you live in the northern part of the country, you may experience depression if there is a lack of adequate exposure to sunlight. All of these conditions have shown to be associated with disturbances in neurotransmitters, the tiny chemical messengers in your brain that have profound effects on your mood, appetite, cravings, sleep, and basic drives, and they are significantly affected by stress.

Serotonin is one of the brain neurotransmitters that has been linked to stress-related symptoms. (The fundamental units of your brain, the neurons or nerve cells, secrete neurotransmitters that transmit messages back and forth from nerves to muscles, glands, or body organs. Neurotransmitters are powerful chemicals that regulate your pain, anxiety, depression, and memory.) The best way to raise or maintain serotonin blood levels is to increase your intake of foods that contain tryptophan. An amino acid found in all foods that are rich in protein—eggs, cheese, milk, fish, meat, poultry, and brown rice—tryptophan is a building block for serotonin, which helps you to go to sleep and makes you feel laid back. Tryptophan has also been shown to benefit migraine sufferers and relieve depression and was formerly a popular supplement to improve sleep. However, all such products were withdrawn because problems in the manufacturing process abroad led to serious illness and fatalities.

Some of the foods highest in this substance are chicken, seafood, turkey, and nuts. Research shows that concentrations of tryptophan and serotonin in the brain can be raised even more when consumption of tryptophan-rich foods is followed by consumption of carbohydrates. So, if you are stressed and having difficulty sleeping, eat one or more of these tryptophan-rich foods and then have a carbohydrate (bread, rice, piece of fruit, etc.) an hour before bedtime.

If you're a vegetarian, just load up on cooked dried beans or peas and eat a slice of bread or have a little rice and you can achieve the same effect. If you don't like that combo, try beans and milk or rice and sunflower seeds. Too much protein can just add to stress, so a little goes a long way. These food combos should put you in dreamland.

USE MONOUNSATURATED OILS TO REDUCE HUNGER PANGS

Monounsaturated oils like olive oil can reduce hunger pangs. The results of one study presented at the Experimental Biology 2000 Conference in San Diego supported this idea. In Specter's study, men were served lunch prepared with either a monounsaturated or polyunsaturated oil mix. Four to eight hours later, those in the monounsaturated group were significantly less hungry than the other group. If you eat a salad or some food with olive oil for lunch, you may reduce the desire for late-afternoon snacks. Monounsaturated oils also help prevent cardiovascular disease and possibly cancer.

EAT EGGS; IT'S OK!

Eggs are good for you, if you're not allergic to them. Egg yolks supply lutein and zeaxanthin, two carotenoids that positively affect vision. In fact, the chicken egg is the standard against which other protein sources are measured. The Net Protein Utilization, or NPU, is the measure of biological value and protein digestibility of foods. The egg is at the top of the NPU list, followed by fish, cheese, brown rice, red meat, and poultry. The fact is, Americans eat too much protein, two to three times the recommended amount. Like any other protein, eggs should be eaten in moderation, but just remember that they are an excellent source of protein and can provide endless eating variety. What other food can you poach, scramble, boil, and use in a souffle and to hold other ingredients together? The egg is supreme. Yes, it contains cholesterol, but it also contains lecithin, a substance that protects against cholesterol. Besides, as we said in chapter 3, it's not the cholesterol that's bad for you; it's the trans-fats. Eggs also contain hefty amounts of B vitamins, the vitamins that protect you against stress. B vitamins also reduce homocysteine, the culprit behind heart and artery disease.

EAT HIGH-ZINC FOODS TO HELP YOU LOSE WEIGHT

The mineral zinc may play a role in body fat regulation and could help you lose weight, according to a study in the *Journal of the American College of Nutrition*. Researchers at Beth Israel Deaconess Medical Center in Boston[11] found that zinc may influence levels of leptin, a hormone that plays a key role in the feedback loop that maintains energy balance. It works by signaling the state of energy stores to the brain and influencing the regulation of appetite and energy metabolism. Leptin can make you feel full even when you're not. This hormone is produced in fat cells and tells you when to eat and when to put down your fork. If you're overweight, you may not produce enough leptin to curb your food cravings. In their study, the researchers discovered that blood levels of leptin increased when sixty milligrams of zinc were added to participants' daily diets. In contrast, men who were fed zinc-deficient diets produced less leptin. Some researchers think that when fat is lost, leptin production decreases, which may explain why dieters regain weight. Maintaining high leptin levels may help you keep weight off once you've lost it. As the study showed, zinc may play a key role in helping keep leptin levels high. Foods that contain zinc include oysters, herring, eggs, nuts, wheat germ, liver, and red meat. If you do decide to increase your zinc intake, remember that dietary fiber, calcium, and foods that contain phytate (dried beans, whole grains, and peanut butter) can interfere with zinc absorption, so go easy on them.

REACHING FOR CHOCOLATE MAY BE A SIGN OF MAGNESIUM DEFICIENCY

Recent research[12] has found that chcolate may be used by some people as a self-medication for dietary deficiencies, especially magnesium. If you crave chocolate and find it is a major pitfall in your effort to lose weight and keep it off, try eating more high-magnesium foods and see if that helps. Foods high in magnesium include whole-grain breads and cereals, fresh peas, brown rice, soy flour, wheat germ, nuts, Swiss chard, figs, green leafy vegetables, and citrus fruits (oranges, tangerines, tangeloes, and grapefruits).

EAT FOODS FULL OF B VITAMINS TO REDUCE YOUR STRESS

The B vitamins are your ticket to stress-free eating. Foods with B vitamins in them do everything from promoting good digestion (including helping you metabolize fatty foods) to dissolving cholesterol and enhancing your mood. In fact, a recent review of the research on the effect of nutrients on mood reported four double-blind studies that showed an improvement in thiamine status (one of the B vitamins) was associated with improved mood.[13]

Inadequate vitamin B_6 status has been associated with altered neuropsychiatric function, possibly due to its effect on the metabolism of serotonin. In one study[14] HIV-positive men showed a significant decline in psychological distress when their vitamin B_6 status was normalized from inadequate to adequate status. In another study[15] women with poor vitamin B_6 concentration in their breast milk had babies who were difficult to console and these mothers were less responsive to their infants' cries.

So, if you're feeling stressed, consider eating more foods with B vitamins in them. Look at the following table for a summary of the B vitamins, their stress-reducing functions, deficiency symptoms or signs, and good food sources.

VITAMIN SOURCES	STRESS-REDUCING FUNCTIONS	DEFICIENCY SYMPTOMS	SOME FOOD SOURCES
B_1 (thiamine)	promotes good digestion, helps with metabolism	fatigue, inability to sleep, overreacting to normal stress, rapid heartbeat, lack of enthusiasm, feeling like going crazy	sunflower seeds, rolled oats, lima beans, soybeans, raisins, wheat germ, peas, whole-wheat-flour foods, asparagus, brown rice
B_2 (riboflavin)	helps metabolize proteins and carbohydrates	feeling trembly, dizzy, sluggish, overly nervous, tiring easily	chicken, peanuts, spinach, kale, brewer's yeast, eggs, peas
B_3 (niacin)	helps in the digestion of carbohydrates and vitamins B_1 and B_2	feeling overly anxious, weak, or tired, memory loss	wheat bran, tuna, turkey, salmon, rabbit

B₆ (pyridoxine)	aids in the metabolism of fats, carbohydrates, protein, potassium, regulates water imbalance, dissolves cholesterol, mood elevator	feeling tense, irritable, or nervous, unable to sleep, puffiness, dermatitis or eczema, bloating, soreness, cramps	white beans, mackerel, liver, sweet potatoes, cooked cabbage, bananas
B₁₂	carbohydrate, fat, and protein metabolism, fertility, resistance to germs	feeling apathetic, moody, forgetful, suspicious, difficulty walking or talking, arm or leg soreness	clams, oysters, sardines, crab, crayfish, trout, herring, sea vegetables (dulse, kombu, kelp, wakame), fermented soyfoods (tempeh, natto, miso)
Folic acid	proper mental functioning, healthy fetuses	looking pale and wan, feeling "pooped," panting with slight exertion	fresh dark green uncooked vegetables
Pantothenic acid	protects against environmental stress, and infection aids in expelling trapped gas, protects	chronic gas or distension, fatigue, balky bowels, strange itching or burning sensations	dark buckwheat, lobster, sweet potatoes, organ meats, eggs, oysters, broccoli, cauliflower,

			sesame seeds
	against side effects of antibiotics, helps produce body energy		
Biotin	helps metabolize fats, proteins, and carbohydrates, maintains skin, hair, nerves, and sebaceous glands	nausea and vomiting, muscle pains, sore mouth and lips, poor appetite	nutritional yeast, liver, mushrooms, lima beans, yogurt, nuts, fish, eggs, beans, grains
Inositol	may control fat metabolism	not known	wheat germ, oranges, grapefruits, nuts, cantaloupes, whole-grain breads and cereals, bulgar, wheat, rice, lima beans, peaches, lettuce, peas, nutritional yeast, molasses
Choline	keeps blood pressure down, helps resistance to infection, essential to nerve conduction, liver function	poor thinking ability	egg yolks, soybeans, liver, fish, peanuts, wheat germ, lecithin

ADAPTED FROM: *Wellness Practitioner*, by Carolyn Chambers Clark, copyrighted by the author, Springer Publishing Company, 1996.

It's easy to see how helpful B vitamins are to food digestion and potentially to weight loss. Now we're going to help you apply this information. On the following pages you'll find some recipes that are chock-full of B vitamins. Remember, those are the vitamins that can help to reduce your stress and metabolize fats, so you'll want to eat plenty of the foods in the preceding table.

WHY USE MONOUNSATURATED FATS?

You'll notice that the recipes that use oil call for olive oil. There is a reason for this. We recommend olive oil because it is fragrant and can be used for both cooking and salads. Fats that are solid at room temperature, such as those found in meat or poultry and butter, are saturated fats. Fats that are "unsaturated" stay liquid at room temperature. Some unsaturated fats are good for you while others aren't. Corn, soybean, and safflower oils and some margarines are mostly polyunsaturated fat, which is the fat that is harmful for your heart, adding extra stress to your body. So, don't eat any of those. Always use a monounsaturated fat for cooking and salad oils. Olive oil is largely monounsaturated and contains the beneficial acid oleic. Not only is olive oil able to lower the "bad" cholesterol and raise the "good" cholesterol, but it also lowers blood pressure, blocks the tendency of blood to clot (protecting against stroke), soothes the stomach, and protects against gallbladder disease (by activating bile flow and raising HDL "good" cholesterol). Olive oil also protects against cellular damage and genetic "errors" that cause cancers and aging. Because olive oil has such a rich taste, a little goes a long way. Use olive oil on vegetables or baked potatoes instead of margarine or butter. It's good for you!

RECIPES—MAIN DISHES

Crunchy Chicken

INGREDIENTS

2 eggs, beaten
2 chicken breasts with the skin removed
$1/2$ cup wheat germ or whole-wheat flour
$1/2$ cup sunflower seeds or finely chopped peanuts
enough olive oil to lightly coat the bottom of a
    baking dish

Mix the beaten eggs with a tablespoon of two of water. Dip the chicken first in the egg mixture, then in the wheat germ or flour, then in the sunflower seeds or peanuts. Lay the chicken in a baking dish that has been coated with olive oil and bake at 375°F for 45 minutes.

Makes 2 portions. Serve with a side order of rice and mushrooms or sweet potatoes (with olive oil) and a big green salad of dandelion, arugula, chickory, or other dark greens and olive oil and cidar vinegar dressing. (Eat the second portion cold the next day over a huge salad of greens with a side order of vegetable or lentil soup.)

Smothered Tempeh

If you're a vegetarian or just want to experience the joys of eating a healthy meal without animal protein, try this tempeh recipe.

INGREDIENTS

8 ounces of tempeh (found at health food stores)
2 cups fresh green peas
2 cups fresh ripe tomatoes, chopped
1 clove garlic, minced
fresh sage, basil, parsley, or oregano to taste
2–4 baked sweet or white potatoes as an accom-
    paniment

$^1/_2$ cup raisins
1 tablespoon of olive oil

Cut the tempeh in strips and stir-fry with the peas, tomatoes, garlic, and spices in olive oil. When tomatoes and peas are just about done, throw in the raisins. Makes 2 servings.

Dr. Clark's Potato and Broccoli Omelette

INGREDIENTS
1 tablespoon of olive oil
1–2 stalks of broccoli, diced
1 diced onion
1 clove garlic
2 baked potatoes, diced
4 eggs, beaten and thinned with a little soy milk
1 tablespoon dulse, miso, or kelp
thinly sliced tomato, cooked asparagus, and/or
    walnuts as garnish

Heat the olive oil in a large skillet and slowly sauté the broccoli, onion, and garlic until tender. Throw in the potatoes and heat until warm. Stir in the eggs and dulse, miso, or kelp. After the eggs start to set, flip one end over so you have a folded-in-half omelette. Place the garnish on top of the omelette and let the omelette cook until all the egg has set. Serve with a salad of greens and a homemade olive oil and cidar vinegar dressing. Makes 2 servings.

Tangy Fish

INGREDIENTS
1 tablespoon of olive oil
2 trout, mackerel, or salmon fillets
one 8-ounce can of cubed pineapple or peaches
    packed in juice

1 tablespoon soy sauce or aminos (without MSG
   or added salt; from health food store)
cornstarch
fresh grated ginger
3–4 cooked prunes, quartered

Preheat the oven to 400°F. Put the olive oil in the bottom
of a Pyrex container and place the fillets flat on the oil.
Turn the fillets over to coat them. Mix the fruit juice with
a little soy sauce and cornstarch and whisk until smooth.
Place a little olive oil in a small sauce- or frying pan and
sauté the ginger gently. Add the fruit and cook gently until it begins to bubble. Add the cornstach mixture and stir
until it thickens. Pour the sauce over the fillets and bake
them for 15–20 minutes or until they flake easily when
poked with a fork. Makes 2 servings.

Snappy Paella with Rice

INGREDIENTS
optional: 1 pound of lobster tails or cultivated
   mussels cleaned of their "beards"
1 cup of brown rice
1 1/2 pounds of cooked shrimp
1 tablespoon of olive oil
2 cloves garlic
1 large onion
1 pound of canned tomatoes or 6 fresh tomatoes
13 ounces of chicken broth (buy without MSG
   from the health food store)
cayenne pepper to taste
1/8 tsp saffron
1 cup fresh or frozen peas

Soak the mussels for an hour in cold water if gritty and
scrub with a stiff brush under running water. Discard any
with cracked or open shells. Parboil the rice in 2 cups of

boiling salted water for 20 minutes and drain. Meanwhile, sauté the shrimp and/or lobster tails lightly in olive oil and remove them from a paella pan or oven pot. Add a little more oil and sauté the garlic, onion, and tomatoes until soft. Add the chicken broth, cayenne, and saffron. Bring the mixture to a boil and spoon it on top of the rice; add the seafood. Bake until rice is tender and most of the liquid has been absorbed, 30–45 minutes, then stir in the peas and seafood. Cover and bake another 10 minutes. Serves 6.

Dr. Clark's Stuffed Squash
If you're feeling adventurous, try this delicious recipe.

INGREDIENTS
2 large yellow squash, halved and partially scooped out
2 cloves garlic, peeled and crushed
1 tablespoon of olive oil
1/2 onion, minced
1 cup cooked brown rice
1 tablespoon of wheat germ
4 ounces cubed tempeh
fresh (or dried) thyme, rosemary, and/or basil
12 ounces of V8 or tomato juice or stewed tomatoes
handful raw chopped peanuts or grated soy cheese

Sauté the scooped-out squash with the garlic. Pour the oil into a large flat casserole or roasting pan. In a bowl, mix together all the other ingredients except the tomato juice or stewed tomatoes and the peanuts or soy cheese. Stuff the squash with the mixture, mounding it to fit. Pour the tomato juice or tomatoes over the squash. Sprinkle with soy cheese or grated peanuts and additional herbs and bake in a preheated 375°F oven for 45 minutes or until the squash is tender. For variety, use raisins instead of peanuts or soy cheese or experiment with using other high-B-vitamin foods.

Although the next two recipes aren't especially strong in B vitamins, they have other stress-reducing benefits. You'll find the explanation at the end of each recipe.

All-Week-Long Tomato Sauce
Make on Saturday or Sunday and then use all week long.[1]

Coat the bottom of a large *iron pot* with extra-virgin olive oil. Cut up to a size that suits you and then gently sauté the following:

1 large onion
1–3 cloves of garlic, to taste
3 green, red, or yellow peppers
1–2 cans of artichoke hearts, drained
1 handful fresh or home-dried *basil*
1 handful fresh or home-dried *oregano*
1 large 15-ounce can crushed *tomatoes*
1 large 15-ounce can tomato puree
1–2 6-ounce cans tomato paste

Cover and let simmer on low for 20–50 minutes, stirring occasionally to prevent sticking. Use this versatile sauce all week long: scoop large spoonfuls onto baked potatoes, rice, pasta, steamed vegetables, or salad. For variety, add fat-free ground beef substitute from the health food store, cubed tofu or tempeh, or additional steamed vegetables. For even more verve, sprinkle on Modern Products Naturally Cajun seasoning (find it at your health food store). Every meal will be tasty, filling, and good for you, too!

EXPLANATION OF INGREDIENTS:
If you're a woman, use an *iron pot*. Many women are iron-depleted and feel fatigued and stressed because of

it.[13] Iron depletion also leads to poor memory and poor verbal learning.

Though studies[14,15,16] have found differing results about other benefits of higher iron intake, it does seem clear that the type of iron derived from cooking in iron pots, nonheme iron, may provide greater benefit with less risk than iron derived from eating meat. The bottom line: cooking in iron pots is an easy way to provide nonheme iron if you're a woman.

Use fresh *oregano* and *basil*—even better, grow it yourself! Having an herb garden is a real stress-reducer. The thrill of watching something grow is a marvelous antidote to daily anxiety. Start with a small kitchen herb garden and progress to growing greens and small vegetables in pots or in a garden. It's great therapy for the soul.

Tomatoes have lycopene, which protects against heart disease and prostate cancer, and vitamin C, an antioxidant that deals with stressful free radicals.

Dr. Clark's Power Salad

Eat some variety of this salad every day. When you can, serve with a cup or bowl of pea, bean, or lentil soup for extra protein and fiber. If you work, make 5 batches of salads over the weekend and place them in well-sealed plastic containers in your refrigerator. Take one with you each day with a side order of tomato sauce, *homemade* oil and vinegar dressing, or oil and lemon juice and a shaker of Cajun seasoning, as well as an attractive bowl to eat from. When eating at home, also use a large bowl or plate that you especially like. Never eat out of plastic or paper containers or directly from the refrigerator.

Arrange a mixture of seasonal *greens,* such as arugula, watercress, beet tops, spinach, escarole, and kale. Experiment, and learn to love the rich taste of dark greens. Try to remember this role of thumb: the darker green the leaf, the more healthy it is. Avoid non-nutritious iceberg lettuce.

Add any of the following vegetables and vary often to reduce the stress of boredom:

- grape tomatoes
- tomato wedges
- green beans
- steamed and cooled artichoke hearts or canned but not marinated artichokes
- cubed baked potatoes
- carrot peelings
- chopped celery
- black olive
- pumpkin, sunflower, sesame, or flax seeds
- pickles
- radishes

Make sure you add one of these each day to ensure you have enough protein:

- cubes of tofu
- boiled sliced egg
- refried nonfat beans with rice crackers or cooked rice

When not adding potatoes to your salad, chew on a few vegetable rice crackers dabbed with peanut butter for extra flavor and energy.

EXPLANATION OF INGREDIENTS
Homemade dressing is more healthful, as bottled salad dressings are full of stressful artificial ingredients and almost always contain sugar.

Not only will the salad *greens* help rebuild cells stressed by free radicals, but also the fiber in the vegetables helps promote weight loss, relieve constipation, prevent colon cancer, and release carcinogens and toxins from the intestinal tract.

Consider growing your own organic *greens* for a double treat when you eat them. Not only will your salads be pesticide-free and less stressful for your digestive tract and entire body, but also you can chew with pride in your accomplishment.

USING NATURAL SWEETENERS

Slowly introduce your body to natural sweeteners. While sugar can drain and stress you, stevia, carob (both available at health food stores), and other natural sweeteners, including raisins, pineapple, dates, prunes, and bananas, can give you energy. You can also use vanilla and cinnamon to satisfy your sweet tooth. For high energy as well as a sweet treat, mix up some of Dr. Clark's High Energy Breakfast Drink.

Dr. Clark's High-Energy Breakfast Drink

MIX IN A BLENDER:
1 tablespoon *carob* powder
1 tablespoon *soy powder*
1 heaping teaspoon *flax seeds* (or blend them by
    themselves into into a nutty-tasting powder)
6–8 ounces *pineapple juice*
1 tablespoon liquid *lecithin*

WHEN SMOOTH ADD:
8–10 frozen strawberries (add 1 or 2 at a time)
or
1 quartered banana

Don't blend the fruit all the way; leave some of it in small chunks. Enjoy, chewing each mouthful fully, savor the chocolaty flavor and the crunchy sensations.

EXPLANATION OF INGREDIENTS

Carob is a naturally sweet substance that helps relax a stressed digestive tract.

Soy powder packs a wallop in the protein department and keeps the hormones balanced to create a feeling of calm.

Flax seeds are one of the most potent sources of "good fats," as well as being a highly digestible source of protein. They are packed with essential fatty acids for alert brain activity and powerful antioxidants for destressing the body.

Pineapple juice is naturally sweet, full of digestive enzymes, and packed with vitamin C, an antioxidant that will derail stressful free radicals.

Lecithin is another soybean product that lowers blood cholesterol, lessens the risk of heart disease, improves brain function, promotes energy, and helps repair liver damage. It is needed by the whole body. Cell membranes that regulate the passage of nutrients in and out of cells are largely composed of lecithin. Finally, lecithin is a great emulsifying agent and will give any drink a wonderful consistency.

Sinfully Good Pumpkin

Try some sinfully good pumpkin if you have a sweet tooth. Add a little mashed tofu and 2–3 custard cups of the pumpkin could be your dinner! The 20-ounce can makes about 12 custard cups, so save the rest in the refrigerator for when your sweet tooth acts up.

INGREDIENTS
1 tablespoon of olive oil
1 20-ounce can of pumpkin
1 16-ounce container of soy milk (experiment with organic original, vanilla, and carob)
2 eggs

cinnamon, ground ginger, cardomom, and/or
cloves

optional: 1 ounce real maple syrup (not the imita-
tion kind)

Rub a little olive oil around the bottom and sides of a
dozen small custard cups. Mix the pumpkin with the container of soy milk, eggs, and spices. Pour into the custard
cups and bake for 15 minutes at 425°F. Reduce the oven
temperature to 350°F for 40–50 minutes, until a knife in-
serted into the center comes back clean. Cool and serve.
Add maple syrup if desired. Eat two or three for dinner
and keep the rest in your fridge for when you need a
sweet treat.

START YOUR HEALTHY FOOD PLAN TODAY

Now that you have some good ideas about what kinds of
foods are going to help you lose weight, be sure to make
a contract with yourself to begin eating more of these
foods and take pride in the fact that you are eating to stay
well.

Pick a Goal for This Week and the Next

Choose a goal from the following list for this week and
then choose one for next week, too.

Decide which one has the most value to you and go for
it!

___ I will eat breakfast every day, starting tomorrow.

___ I will cook my food and enjoy the process and
creativity of it all.

___ Starting tomorrow, I will eat more veggies,
fruits, and raw nuts.

___ By the end of this week I will eat more high-
satisfaction foods.

___ Within three days I will start eating more high-vitamin-B foods.

___ By the end of this week I will switch to a natural sweetener or stop using sweetener altogether.

___ By tomorrow, I will eat my biggest meal in the morning and my smallest meal at night.

___ I will drink eight glasses of water every day.

REFERENCES

1. Benardot, D., R. C. Deutz, D. E. Martin, and M. M. Cody. 2000. Relationship between energy deficits and body composition in elite female gymnasts and runners. *Medicine and Science in Sports and Exercise* 32(3): 659–68.

2. Bergogne-Berezin, E., P. Courvalin, P. Gehanno, J. Demaresy, C. Perrone, and R. Ducluzeau. 1998. Forum on bacterial resistance. *Presse Medicine* 27(35): 1796–1800.

3. File, T. M. 1999. Overview of resistance in the 1990s. *Chest* 115(Supplement 3): 3S–8S.

4. Morgan, W. A., and B. J. Clayshute. 2000. Pecans lower low-density lipoprotein cholesterol in people with normal lipid levels. *Journal of the American Dietetic Association* 100(3): 312–18.

5. Fraser, E. 1999. Nut consumption, lipids and risk of a coronary event. *Clinical Cardiology* 22(Supplement 7): III: 11–15.

6. Edwards, S., I. Kwaw, J. Matud, and I. Kurtz. 1999. Effect of pistachio nuts on serum lipid levels in patients' moderate hypercholesteremia. *Journal of the American College of Nutrition* 18(3): 229–32.

7. Hu, F. B., M. J. Stampfer, J. E. Manson, E. B. Rimm, G. A. Colditz, B. A. Rosner, F. E. Speizer, C. H. Hennekas, and W. C. Willett. 1998. Frequent nut consumption and risk of coronary heart disease in women: Prospective cohort study. *British Medical Journal* 317(7169): 1341–45.

8. Feldman, L. E. M. 1985. Serotonin content of foods: Effect on urinary excretion of 5-hydroxyendoleacetic acid. *American Journal of Clinical Nutrition* 42(4): 639–43.

9. Rolls, B. J., and D. L. Miller. 1997. Is the low-fat message

giving people a license to eat more? *Journal of the American College of Nutrition* 16(6): 535–43.

10. Maciejko, J. J., R. Braz, A. Shah, S. Patil, and M. Rubenfire. 1994. Psyllium for the reduction of cholestyramine-associated gastrointestinal symptoms in the treatment of primary hypercholesterolemia. *Archives of Family Medicine* 3(11): 955–60.

11. Mantzoros, C. S., A. S. Prasad, F. W. Beck, S. Grabowski, J. Kaplan, C. Adair, and G. J. Brewer. 1998. Zinc may regulate serum leptin concentrations in humans. *Journal of the American College of Nutrition* 17: 270–75.

12. Bruinsma, K., and D. L. Taren. 1999. Chocolate: Food or drug? *Journal of the American Dietetic Association* 99(10): 1249–56.

13. Benton, D., and R. T. Donohoe. 1999. The effects of nutrients on mood. *Public Health Nutrition* 2(3A): 403–9.

14. Tuomainen, T. P., K. Punnonen, K. I. Nyyssonene, and J. T. Salonen. 1998. Association between body iron stores and the risk of acute myocardial infarction in men. *Circulation* 97(15): 1461–66.

15. Klipstein-Grobusch, K., D. E. Grobbee, J. H. den Breeijen, H. Boeing, A. Hofman, and J. C. Witteman. 1999. Dietary iron and risk of myocardial infarction in the Rotterdam Study. *American Journal of Epidemiology* 149(5): 412–418.

CHAPTER 5

Step 4: Train Your Stress Response to Stop Binge Eating

Pam, a school principal, told us: "I have a very stressful job. When I get home, I make dinner for everyone else. By that time, I'm exhausted. When no one's around, I take down a gallon of ice cream or a big bag of potato chips and hide in the bedroom or laundry room, eating. I'm not really hungry, but when I'm chewing, I can forget all the bad things that happened to me that day. Before I even realize it, I've eaten all the ice cream or chips. Yes, I'm overweight, more than fifty pounds overweight, and I don't feel like having sex anymore or talking to my friends or dealing with my teenage children. I'm depressed, but who wouldn't be down given the way I look and feel?"

Jim, a part-time computer salesman, told us: "When I was a kid, my mother used to put a plate of cookies in front of me and then call me fat and send me to bed without dinner when I ate them all. I started dieting in high school to lose weight and I've been thin and I've been fat over the years. I've been steadily gaining weight again since I lost my job two years ago. I found two part-time jobs that keep me running day and night, but they don't give me enough money. I don't see my friends anymore and spend all my free time on the Internet with a six-pack and whatever snacks I can find. Once I start eating, I can't stop. This whole thing is all my fault. If I hadn't lost my job, I probably wouldn't be in this mess."

Pam and Jim are victims of binge eating. They are stressed and they turn to food to help them. Food may give them the one pleasure they allow themselves. They're not alone. For many people, maybe even you, binge eating provides a temporary distraction from problems and can temporarily reduce stress and be soothing.

If you binge, you may not even think about your hunger and may not even remember the taste of what's been eaten. You may have lost the ability to tell when you're really hungry. Food is there and it's comforting, so you eat.

SEROTONIN AND BINGING

Binges may be driven by the need to increase serotonin, a feel-good brain chemical that can help relax and calm you. Eating carbohydrates increases serotonin levels, while eating protein reduces them. (If this is true for you, being on a high-protein/high-fat diet will lead to binging quicker than anything else. However, you probably have noticed that when you eat pasta, bread, and chocolate you feel soothed and relaxed.)

Your brain may not be producing enough serotonin and food may become your drug of choice for reducing anxiety and depression. It could also be that you enjoy the way carbohydrates change your mood. Helen, a forty-two-year-old administrative assistant, felt that way:

Chocolate calms me like nothing else. I feel drowsy and relaxed when I have a candy bar, and it doesn't matter anymore if my boss is yelling at me for this or that report. I hate to tell you this, but I think I'm addicted to the stuff.

HOW INSULIN PLAYS A ROLE IN BINGE EATING

Insulin can be produced just by thinking about eating or seeing food. When this happens, your blood glucose is lowered and a food binge may seem like the right response. Instead, it's important to stop and pay attention to your internal hunger and spend less time thinking about food and what to eat. The best way to start becoming aware of internal hunger is to start a Binge Journal. A sample Binge Journal for Joyce, a thirty-year-old computer programmer, appears here. Joyce often tried to lose weight by severely limiting her food intake, to 600 calories a day. To do that, she skipped breakfast and had a canned diet drink for lunch and dinner.

Here is a portion of Joyce's Binge Journal:

Friday, January 28, 2000
I have been keeping on my diet for a week, but today I weakened. I had to give my office mate a ride home after work. She is not an easy person to get along with and I have to bite my tongue to keep from shouting at her. After I dropped her off, I was already late for my dinner and I was starving. I drove by an ice-cream store, stopped, and bought a gallon of chocolate chocolate chip. I ate the whole thing in my car outside the shop, then threw the carton in the garbage so my husband wouldn't see it and question me about it. On the way home, I shouted at myself for being so stupid. I felt so out of control and depressed. Why can't I stop this stupid behavior? I was off my diet the whole weekend and gained five pounds. I feel so upset and discouraged. What's the use? I may as well accept the fact that I'll be overweight for the rest of my life.

If you binge-eat, we suggest you start a Binge Journal. Purchase a notebook or journal to use only to write about your binge-eating experiences. Make sure you choose the type of notebook or journal that appeals to you—one that will encourage you to write in it every day. Include the trigger experiences that precede your binge eating as well as your thoughts and feelings before, during, and after your binge. Look for patterns and situations that set you up to binge.

YOUR FEELINGS AND BINGING

As the studies we've cited have shown, feelings of stress and anxiety often lead to overeating. The most common feelings leading to binge eating are anger, anxiety, depression, shame, and boredom. This is what happened to Joyce. The worse she felt about herself and the stronger her feelings were, the more she binged.

The urge to binge often comes about during periods of being overly hungry, fatigued, hungover, lonely, in conflict with someone, in an unsatisfying relationship, feeling coerced or manipulated at work or home, or not being able to relax, have fun, and enjoy life. Another major source of binge eating is the desire to escape from the painful emotions that result from not meeting someone else's high standards or ideals.

Any of these situations can lead to binging, making it more difficult to stick with a weight loss plan. Controlling appetite may be the most important part of not binging. It can also be the most difficult. Self-regulation is the process responsible for stopping irresistible impulses, such as food cravings. Remember, you don't have to act on your impulse. Count to ten; distract yourself by reading a favorite book, exercising, getting a hug or massage, or doing some other nurturing activity.

Controlling the urge to binge is going to be a lot harder if you are fatigued, it's late at night, or a situation seems to demand a certain kind of behavior, such as when your friends or family exert pressure for you to overeat.

A nice thing about training your stress response is that

the strength of your control can increase over time. Just as physical exercise can strengthen flabby muscles, conscious self-regulation can help you control irresistible urges, and that's what we'll work on next.

Even if your weight loss goals aren't met every day, it's important to keep a positive attitude and, if necessary, forgive yourself. It's OK to break an oath to eat only healthy foods and have a slice or two of chocolate cake or a big dish of ice cream. Just resolve to stick with the goal at the next meal or the next day and do it. Permanent weight loss belongs to the persistent. It's keeping on that counts, not that a pound or two is lost. Consider this a lifelong goal for greater success.

Avoid eating one big meal a day and passing up breakfast and lunch—a prescription for evening binging. When eating only one meal a day, the body may go into semi-starvation mode, making it difficult to pass up food. Loss of control over food is mainly dependent on dieting and on a preoccupation with food and/or body shape. Give up trying for control over food and you will begin to lose weight. The body needs regular food and nutrients, not once-a-day feeding. Don't expect to lose the weight you've gained over time overnight. Be patient. Losing weight too fast is too stressful for the body and can cause other problems, so just take it easy.

ARE YOU READY FOR A NONBINGE LIFE?
The road to overcoming binging is a challenging one. Before beginning this journey, you must evaluate your readiness to change.

"GOOD-BYE, BINGE EATING!" QUESTIONNAIRE

Answer each of the questions below with a yes or a no. Count up your yesses. See the information at the end of the questionnaire to interpret your results.

_____ 1. I use binge eating to help me manage my feelings.

_____ 2. Binge eating is an enjoyable recreational activity that keeps me from being bored.

_____ 3. Keeping food to binge on gives me a feeling of comfort and security.

_____ 4. Certain foods soothe and relax me.

_____ 5. Although I hate how I feel after I binge, I resent having to give up binging.

_____ 6. Food is in the top three things that bring me the most emotional or physical pleasure.

_____ 7. I realize that not binge eating means taking control of my life.

_____ 8. I believe that when I give up binge eating I will not only get rid of the negative things like low self-esteem and frustration, but my life will change for the better in other ways, too.

_____ 9. Even though I am giving up binge eating, I believe I will gain freedom from my dependence on food.

_____ 10. I'm tired of living my life from day to day, and I want to decide the kind of life I really want.

_____ 11. There is more to life than being alone and eating.

_____ 12. I'm ready to stop avoiding eating for long periods of time.

_____ 13. I'm ready to stop restricting my calories.

_____ 14. I'm ready to eat "forbidden" foods.

The more yesses you have, the more ready you are to stop binge eating. Even if you have a few nos you may be successful in stopping binge eating. If you have more than 2 or

3 nos you may not be successful in stopping binge eating until you change your attitude. In that case, you might want to stop reading this book and seek counseling specifically focused on elevating your self-esteem.

TAKING CONTROL OF BINGE EATING

The first thing to remember about binge eating is that you're in control. Sometimes it may not seem like it, but let's take a look at some common life situations and see who's really in control.

YOU ARE IN CONTROL!

For each of the following behaviors, check whether You or Someone Else is in control.

BEHAVIORS	YOU'RE IN CONTROL	SOMEONE ELSE IS IN CONTROL
Getting up in the morning	____	____
Brushing your teeth	____	____
Choosing what to wear	____	____
Reading a street sign	____	____
Getting to work/school	____	____
Smoking	____	____
Drinking	____	____
Exercising	____	____
Reading the newspaper	____	____
Paying your bills	____	____
Deciding what to say	____	____
Taking drugs	____	____
Eating	____	____

See? There are a lot of things you are in control of. Granted, other people may influence you to some degree, but for the most part, you have a lot of control over what happens to you. Gaining self-control is a process and a skill, just like learning a new language or mastering the computer. This process has phases. That's good to know, because it means you don't have to do it all at once. You can work into it. The first step is making a commitment.

Make a Commitment to Stop Binge Eating

To stop binge eating, be willing to set goals. That means committing to something specific.

Here is an example of a specific goal: I will write down all the food I eat every day for a week.

Here is an example of a general goal: I will try my best to stop binge eating.

Which of these goals do you think will help you stop binging? If you picked the first goal, you're right! Lots of research has shown that the more specific your goal, the better the result. Why is that? Because you know exactly what you have to do and you know when you've done it—you can take pride in knowing you've done a good job.

It's also wise to set an easy goal when you're first trying something new or difficult. Stopping binge eating certainly falls in the category of doing something difficult. To start, you might set one of the goals that follow. Put a check in front of the one that sounds the best to you and make it your goal this week. Then, write it down on three-by-five cards and tape one to your refrigerator, one to your bathroom mirror, another to your steering wheel, and another to your desk or work space. Notice, we've built in some positive words of encouragement to help you meet your goal. Getting positive support for your goal will make it easier for you to achieve it. Here are the goals:

___ It's getting easier and easier for me to eat three full meals a day, starting with breakfast.

___ I'm finding it easy to sit down at the table with someone else whenever I eat.

___ Today I will drink a full glass of water and enjoy
it before I reach for a snack.
___ I'm finding it easier and easier to say no to food
when I'm not hungry.

If you like, create your own positive goal statement.
Try it out for a couple of days. If you don't like it, choose
another. Remember, you're in control!

Have a Dialogue with Your Food

The next thing we're going to ask you to do to help control your stress response is start a *dialogue about food*
with yourself prior to eating anything, especially if binge
eating is a problem. To gain control over your binging,
you must develop a sense of awareness of how you are
eating, why, and in what circumstances.

DIALOGUE ABOUT FOOD

This dialogue is simple and direct and consists of only
three questions. Before you eat something, engage in a
dialogue with yourself to establish whether (1) you are
hungry or are having other feelings, (2) you are confusing
negative feelings with hunger signals from your body,
and (3) this is the food that is right for you now. Just follow along and answer each question:

STEP 1. AM I REALLY HUNGRY?
Am I hungry now, or am I

___ anxious
___ angry
___ in need of comfort
___ embarrassed
___ some other feeling. Try to identify what it is
here:_____

STEP 2. REDUCE NEGATIVE FEELINGS FIRST. (If feelings are not interfering, go on to Step 3.)

If feelings are interfering and you're really not hungry, you need to reduce the negative feelings you're having before you eat. By engaging in a stress-reduction activity, such as taking a walk, meditating, doing deep-breathing, or whatever procedure you choose, you may find that your need for the food has disappeared. You are reprogramming your hunger signal apparatus. Soon you will know exactly what to eat and when. Box 1 shows you how to deep-breathe until you feel relaxed and ready to go on. Box 2 provides a meditation you can do to reduce negative feeling and enhance personal power. Box 3 demonstrates a relaxation procedure that can help you reduce negative feelings. Try at least one of them. Better yet, try two or more different methods. By learning these methods, you will be learning valuable information you can use in other tense situations. Go on to Step 3 if you still want the food after completing at least one stress-reduction procedure.

BOX 1— LEARNING TO DEEP-BREATHE

When upset, you probably breathe in the upper part of your chest. Anger, fear, anxiety, tension, shame, and other negative feelings are in control when you breathe in the upper part of your chest. Follow the directions below to change to deep and relaxing breathing. If you can, find a calm someone to read these directions to you. If you can't, consider recording them into a tape recorder and playing it back. Be sure to read the directions in your most calm and soothing voice:

1. Find a quiet and peaceful spot. If you like, turn on some calming music.

2. Kick off your shoes and loosen any restrictive clothing.

3. Lie or sit down in a comfortable spot.

4. Place one hand on your abdomen.

BOX 1— LEARNING TO DEEP-BREATHE (CONT.)

5. Close your eyes and gently suggest to your body to push your hand out and let your abdomen rise as you breathe in.

6. Exhale, feeling your abdomen retract.

7. When you're ready, inhale again, keeping your hand on your abdomen.

8. Keep breathing in and out in a relaxed manner, letting your hand go in and out with your abdomen. Experience how calm you are becoming.

BOX 2—MEDITATION TO STOP BINGING

1. Breathe in and out and say to yourself on the inhale, "I am in control of what I eat."

2. Breathe out and say to yourself on the exhale, "I eat only what I need to eat to stay healthy."

3. Continue breathing in and saying, "I am in control of what I eat," and breathing out saying "I eat only what I need to eat to stay healthy."

Alternative statements:

"I am breathing in calm and control."

"I am breathing out worry and fear."

BOX 3—RELAXING TO REDUCE NEGATIVE FEELINGS

Using a calm, soothing voice, read these direcions into a tape recorder and play them back. Be sure to pause after each sentence, just taking your time and reading the directions in a slow, soothing voice:

1. Find a quiet and peaceful spot.

2. Kick off your shoes and loosen any restrictive clothing.

BOX 3—RELAXING TO REDUCE NEGATIVE FEELINGS (CONT.)

3. Lie or sit down in a comfortable spot.

4. Close your eyes and focus your attention on the tape.

5. Think about how slow and relaxed your breathing is getting.

6. Notice how as you breathe in and out you are getting more and more relaxed.

7. Feel the sensations of your body relaxing into the bed or chair.

8. If any thoughts come to mind, let them just drift away.

9. If the thoughts persist, put a mental label on them of the time you will return to these thoughts. For now, you are just breathing easily . . . drifting . . . relaxing.

10. Focus your attention on your left foot. Notice how heavy and relaxed it is becoming.

11. The next time you inhale, send a wave of relaxation to your left foot.

12. The next time you inhale, send that wave of relaxation up your left foot and up your left leg.

13. The next time you inhale, send that wave of relaxation from your left foot up your left leg and all the way up the rest of your body, letting it flow out the top of your head.

14. Now focus your attention on your right foot. Notice how heavy and relaxed it is becoming.

15. The next time you inhale, send a wave of relaxation up your right foot and up your right leg.

16. The next time you inhale, send that wave of relaxation up both your feet and all through your body, letting it flow down your arms and out your fingertips as you exhale.

17. Keep breathing and letting the relaxation flow through you, just enjoying the wonderfully calm and comforting feelings you are having.

When you feel totally relaxed, you are ready to go to Step 3.

STEP 3. IS THIS THE FOOD I REALLY WANT AND NEED?

If I am hungry, what kind of food do I really want?

- Picture the food and ask yourself:

  - What color is it?
  - What shape is it?
  - How is the food arranged on the plate or in the container?
  - How much food is there?
  - How big of a portion do I want?

- See yourself tasting the food. Watch yourself swallow the food, and see your digestive tract digesting the food. For each step, experience how that food makes you feel.

- Next, picture how you will feel right after:

  - eating the food
  - fifteen minutes later
  - an hour later
  - a day later
  - next week

If the food seems right for you based on this assessment, get the food. If you still want the food, you should have it, but before you do,

1. Make sure you put the food on a pretty plate.
2. Sit down to eat it slowly and in a pleasant place.
3. Concentrate only on the taste of the food and your enjoyment of it.
4. Enjoy it thoroughly, knowing that it is right for you at this time.

Realize Negative Thoughts May Be Fueling Your Binges

If you binge when stressed, it may be because you are listening to negative ideas you're telling yourself. Thoughts are negative when they put you down, make fun of you, or try to make you feel bad. Begin to pay attention to the kinds of things you tell yourself. Find out if you are critical, telling yourself what you or somebody else did wrong. *It's all my fault* and *It's my mother's fault I'm overweight; she's the one who made me eat all those cookies when I was little* are examples of negative thoughts you may be telling yourself.

So is, *Something bad is going to happen.* That thought can keep you from losing weight because it makes you afraid to try something new for fear it will turn out badly. Maybe your thoughts tease you, making fun of you when you try to eat healthy foods. Maybe your stressful thoughts are about eating nothing or almost nothing all day and then binging on chips and cookies when you're alone.

Maybe you tell yourself to have willpower and to deprive yourself of all the foods that taste good to you. As tension builds up because you want the foods you've forbidden yourself, a binge is inevitable. So is the guilt, more deprivation, and, finally, another binge.

Maybe you tell yourself to just stop eating. But starvation can lead to mood swings and obsessive thoughts about food and eating. You may even stress yourself out, exercising too much, giving you a false sense of energy from the endorphins workouts create. These little "feel-good" substances your brain creates may suppress your appetite, but they don't last long. Prepare yourself for a hunger binge.

Another kind of stress binge occurs when you feel overwhelmed by daily events. Eating can help you numb yourself and distract you from things that upset you. The trouble with using food to calm you down is that it only works for a little while; then the stress returns.

As stressful as overwhelming occurrences are, lack of pleasure is stressful, too. If you have few sources of pleasure in your life, eating may provide an alternative to this humdrum life. Do you ever feel excited about the idea of planning and fantasizing about your next binge? Don't let these fantasies become the focus because your life is unsatisfying in other ways. Change your life if you don't like it. You have the power!

Maybe your binges are fueled by anger. They may be a way of venting your hostility. You could be angry at yourself for anything from making bad investments to being too passive at work—or even for binging. Maybe you're angry at another person. Harris, a young man who came for counseling, felt unappreciated by his wife and overlooked by his supervisor whenever promotions were handed out. He binged when he felt especially mistreated. His binges had a "take that" flavor. Others have told us they were angry at their bodies because they felt let down by their overweight. If you've been abused earlier in life, you may have a lot of anger that you hope food will cure. If you feel as if you've been let down, overlooked, or mistreated or failed at anything, that could be a signal to binge. Just remember, after you've binged, you'll probably feel worse, so instead of jumping into that trap, tell youself: "I'm not going to allow myself to binge. It just isn't worth it."

Another source of binging is habit. Ruth and Jake were victims of habit binging. They ate all day long, eating a reasonable breakfast, then stopping for a second meal on the way to work and a dinner after work before they went home and ate another meal. At work, they kept drawers full of candy bars and potato chips for afternoon snacks.

It's clear there are many sources of binge eating.[1,2,3,4,5,6] Whatever your source is, let's take a look at the next section for ideas about how to reduce binging behavior.

TIPS TO STOP BINGE EATING

Stress is usually a major factor in binge eating. You feel deprived and stressed because you're on a diet. When you can't stand it anymore, you binge. By the time you get to that state of stress, chances are you're not thinking about eating something healthy. You may not be paying attention to how the food tastes or what you're eating. You may even be using food as an escape from the demands and stress of your life. Take note. There are better ways to deal with that stress. More about that later. For now, here are some ways to stop binging forever!

Take these steps to stop binge eating:

1. Challenge your ideas about restricting foods and skipping meals. Every time you catch yourself having these thoughts, tell yourself to "STOP" and picture a big red stop sign. Since emotions and actions follow your thoughts, the sooner you can stop such restrictive dieting ideas from being completed, the less likely you will be to binge.

2. Learn the gentle art of forgiveness if your binges are motivated by anger at yourself or someone else. Underneath the anger you feel is often a deep shame (*What did I do to deserve this?*) and a sense of moral failure (*Why me?*). Make a list of everyone you feel has wronged you. Make sure your name is on that list if you think you've failed at anything. You will need to restore your faith in your own and others' worthiness and accept the myth of a fair and just world to stop these binges. Try some of the stress management suggestions later in this chapter, but keep in mind that you may want to consult a therapist or spiritual adviser if you need additional support.

3. Allow yourself to eat all foods in moderation.

No food is either good or bad, unless you are allergic to it, and those foods you should avoid. You may choose to eat foods that are more healthful, but remember it's your choice. Just like it's your choice to eat foods that may not be so healthful. Legalize foods you've forbidden yourself. Eat at least a portion of one of your "forbidden foods" at least once a week and allow yourself to enjoy it. While eating it, tell yourself, "I deserve to enjoy this food," and then savor every bite. (A portion is one large or three small cookies, one doughnut, or one medium candy bar. For processed foods like ice cream or potato chips, look on the container; it will tell you what an average serving is. Have that.)

4. Make sure you eat enough protein. Protein is composed of amino acids that are essential for production of neurotransmitters, the messengers that signal whether you're hungry or full. Small protein-rich snacks can help you eliminate cravings by keeping your blood sugar and energy levels balanced. Once these snacks are eaten, the message will go to your brain: *I'm full and satisfied. I don't have to eat any more.* If you're worried about binging, carry your snacks with you. What are small protein-rich snacks? Here are some examples, but be creative:

   • A couple of crackers with cheese or peanut butter on them
   • A hard-boiled egg
   • A couple of slices of chicken or turkey
     . . . Get the idea?

5. Eat enough fiber. That means whole-grain cereals, fruits, vegetables, dried beans, whole-grain breads, nuts, and seeds. Fiber slows the

movement of food from your stomach to your small intestine. It creates a feeling of fullness, making it easier to limit your intake of food. It also takes more body energy to absorb and digest high-fiber foods than it does to absorb and digest low-fiber foods, so while you're eating you're burning calories.

6. Drink a small amount of unsweetened fruit juice about an hour before you're likely to binge. You'll know when that is. It's when you start to crave food.

7. Avoid foods you're sensitive to. Keep a diary of what you eat and how you feel for the next few hours. If you have a reaction (sweat, feel cold, headache, or other symptoms) that comes on quickly and goes away after an hour or two, you may be sensitive to that food.

8. If sugar cravings are what make you binge, eat five or six small meals at spaced intervals. Make sure each meal is high in protein and low in sugary and processed foods.

9. If you crave fatty foods (French fries, burgers, chips), consider taking flaxseed oil to reduce your cravings. It is rich in essential fatty acids that can quell your urge. Walnut and canola oils are also good sources of fatty acids. Put a couple of tablespoons of them on your salads with a little apple cider vinegar and some fresh or dried herbs.

10. If chocolate is your downfall, try eating foods high in magnesium. (See chapter 4 for ideas.)

11. Exercise. (See chapter 6.) Moderate exercise will help your body use insulin more effectively, so you'll be less likely to binge. It also helps you produce endorphins that reduce hunger.

12. Don't bring binge foods into the house. Don't

plan for a time to eat them, and don't buy them. If you live with someone else, say, "Please help me not binge. I'm asking you not to bring any of my binge foods into the house. Will you help me with this?" Don't go away until this person agrees to help.

13. On days when you know you will have the opportunity to binge without any worry of interruption, plan an activity with somebody else. Refuse to set the stage for binging behavior to occur by leaving the physical area where you binge.

14. Plan at least one activity you can engage in when you get bored. Boredom is a frequent cause of binging. Make sure it is a pleasurable nonfood alternative such as getting a massage or a facial, going shopping, visiting a friend, reading a good book, taking a long walk on a sunny day, or developing a hobby you enjoy. When you feel nurtured, your chances of binging will be greatly reduced.

15. Keep a daily record of the food you eat and the circumstances under which you eat. (See chapter 2 for the Food/Stress Diary.) Use it every day to monitor your eating behavior. The diary will bring your binging behavior under conscious control and make it easier to change.

16. Increase involvement with supportive friends and family. It may be time to ask for help from others. If you do, be sure you only ask people who will be supportive, not people who will nag or be critical. A lot of research[7] shows that if you have a supportive peer, you can achieve wellness goals. What is a supportive friend? According to the research findings, it's someone who listens, encourages discussion of

what's bothering you, tells you you're appreci-
ated, points out your progress toward your
goals, tells you you're OK, shares ways of coping, points out your potential, doesn't nag, re-
assures you that you can be honest, asks you
what you do well, talks calmly, helps you sort
out your ideas and put problems in perspective, has a sense of humor and makes goals fun,
shares activities with you and/or role models
how to cope, and provides hugs.

17. If you need a motivational push and can't find
a supportive friend, consider joining Weight
Watchers or Take Off Pounds Sensibly
(TOPS), two programs that provide good information and support at a reasonable cost. If
these don't work for you, find an expert in behavior change who can help you set goals and
stay focused.

18. Focus only on the days you meet your goal. If
you slip, let it go. When keeping track keep reminding yourself of the positive things you've
done. Give yourself a reward each day you
meet your goal, even if it's something small like
watching a favorite video or calling a good
friend.

19. Picture yourself meeting your goal. Research
shows that by using imagery to picture a positive performance, you are more likely to perform
well. The last thing before you go to bed at
night and the first thing when you get up in the
morning, picture yourself beating the urge to
binge and feeling good about it.

20. Picture yourself fitting into the clothes you like
and feeling more comfortable with your body.

21. Only associate eating with your kitchen or dining room table and only with sitting down.
Avoid working, talking, sewing, or any other

non–food eating or preparation activity while sitting around a kitchen or dining room table. Keep all your food in the kitchen. Only carry your meals or protein snacks with you in your car; do not have food at your desk, in the living room, or anywhere else. Do not have snack foods when watching TV or a video or working at a computer or in your room—all notorious for putting on additional weight. When you eat, make eating the only thing you do—don't watch TV, listen to the radio, read, or work.

22. Eat purposefully.

- While cooking, enjoy the color of lightly steamed vegetables or the shape of a grape.
- Pick foods of different colors and shapes and arrange them on a pretty plate.
- Bring your food to the table before sampling it.
- While chewing, focus only on the taste and texture of your food and how good it smells.
- Eat slowly. Many meals are consumed in five minutes or less. Your body needs time to figure out it's full and send the message to your brain to leave the table. Take the time. It will help you stop binging. You're worth the effort.
- Remind yourself that focusing on what you're eating is the key to success in overcoming binging.
- Leave your chair as soon as you have finished eating.

23. Don't eat or drink anything after you finish your dinner and try to eat your last meal no

later than 6:00 P.M. or, at the latest, 7:00 P.M., so your food has adequate time to be digested before you go to bed. Try to do something active after dinner—take a walk, go dancing, or even clean your house. Do something that engages you so you're not thinking about food.

24. If you feel overwhelmed by circumstances in your life, learn some stress-reduction measures and practice them regularly. See the next sections for ideas.

See the following case study for the story of Patty, a courageous woman who conquered her binge eating, just like you can!

The Story of Patty

Patty told me she had been overweight much of her life. She'd tried every new diet program. Each time, she'd lose weight, then gain it back again. Patty was so frustrated, she broke into tears when she began describing all the diets she'd tried. Now, at age forty-eight, she was the heaviest she'd ever been. "Look at me! I weigh 250 pounds!" It was clear she felt depressed about the way she looked in her clothes and had even lost interest in her hobby, making stuffed bears. When her friends or family told her to lose weight, she got angry and told them to "mind your own business!"

While Patty knew she had a problem with binging, she had long ago decided there was no way to stop it once the urge to eat came over her. "I'm addicted to food," she told me. "I just don't have the willpower to resist a chocolate cake or a pizza." When I told her she wouldn't have to give up her favorite foods, just binging on them, she stopped crying.

She agreed to have one slice of chocolate cake and

two slices of pizza before she came to see me at her next visit. I gave her a list of binging tips, and my only suggestion was that she eat the cake and pizza at the table, while sitting in a chair, and that she do it purposefully. The next week, she reported that she'd felt guilty about eating the foods but got over that pretty quickly and was able to eat them slowly, focusing on how each tasted. "This is new to me," she said. "I did what you said. I only bought two slices so I wouldn't be tempted to eat the whole thing."

At her next visit, she reported that she slipped once and had four slices of pizza instead of two and also had two candy bars instead of the one that she'd planned to eat. "I was rushed for time and ate in my car that day and I ate that second candy bar without even tasting it. I got real down on myself, but then I remembered what you said and forgave myself. I was OK for the rest of the week." We worked on time management and planning so she wouldn't be so rushed for time, and she agreed to leave enough time so she wouldn't be rushed.

Over the next six months, Patty reported binging only twice: once when her brother was killed in a car accident and once when her boss shouted at her in front of two customers. Each time she came to see me, I congratulated her on her willpower, and by her sixth visit she said, "I'm getting more and more confident. Maybe I do have willpower!"

A year later, Patty had gradually lost forty-five pounds and told me, "I don't binge anymore. I enjoy my food and the pounds are coming off slowly. You told me that was healthier anyway, so I'm pleased. I just bought a new suit to celebrate the last five pounds I've lost."

STRESS REDUCERS THAT CAN PREVENT BINGE EATING

Look at the Stress column in the following table. Find the kind of stress that leads to your binging. Next, slide your finger across to the Reduce Stress column. Choose one of the methods and then go to the page where directions for that method appear. If your first choice doesn't work, try the next one until you find the best one for you. It's good to learn several kinds of procedures so you'll have a backup in case the first one doesn't work when you're under stress and in danger of binging.

STRESS	REDUCE STRESS
Deadline anxiety	Time management (SEE PAGE 120) Thought stopping (SEE PAGE 119) Disputing negative self-talk (SEE PAGE 114) Coping comments (SEE PAGE 113)
Interviews/evaluations	Assertiveness (SEE PAGE 109) Progressive relaxation (SEE Box 3, PP. 93–95) Coping comments (SEE PAGE 113)
Spouse/date/friend anxiety	Imagery methods (SEE PAGE 115) Affirmations (SEE PAGE 107) Self-massage (SEE PAGE 118)
Anger when around family	Anger control methods (SEE PAGE 108) Imagery methods (SEE PAGE 115) Affirmations (SEE PAGE 107) Disputing negative self-talk (SEE PAGE 114)

Affirmations to Control Stress

Like most other people, you probably evaluate your performance moment-to-moment. At times, you may call yourself stupid or lazy or other negative names you may have learned in your family. This kind of negative self-talk can be very destructive and can lead to binging when you feel bad enough about yourself. We want to help you to start using positive self-talk all the time. One way to do that is by using affirmations. These are words you say, think, or write that encourage you, soothe you, and boost your self-esteem.

Here are some examples of affirmations you can use to reduce stress and and stop binging:

- ☒ I'm getting more and more control over the food I eat.
- ☒ I feel confident about my ability to stop binging.
- ☒ I'm a good person.
- ☒ I can take a deep breath and calm down.

Try writing some positive affirmations here:

_____

_____

_____

Take the ones that appeal to you and write them on three-by-five cards. Carry the cards with you; tape them on mirrors, your refrigerator, and your desk and steering wheel to give you positive feedback throughout the day.

Anger Control Methods
If anger gets in the way of your staying on your food plan, use one of these methods to feel better and get your focus back.

METHOD 1
1. Close your eyes and identify where anger re-
   sides inside you. Is it in your heart? Your stomach? Your back? Your brain? Someplace else?
2. Collect all the anger from wherever it is in your
   body.
3. Using your imagination, put it in an imaginary
   container.
4. Close the lid of the container.
5. Lock the container and throw away the key.
6. Send it somewhere far, far away where it can no
   longer influence you.

METHOD 2
1. Close your eyes.
2. Turn your anger into a color.
3. Turn your colored anger into a liquid.
4. Let all the anger drain out of your fingers and
   toes.
5. Let the anger drain onto the floor, out the door,
   and far, far away.

Assertiveness

Assertiveness includes speaking up for yourself and your
rights in a way that respects the other person. Whenever
someone attempts to take advantage of you or treats you
disrespectfully, assertive behavior does not guarantee that
the other person will respect your rights, but it will help
you feel good about yourself.

Before you attempt to be assertive, you have to grapple
with the risks of doing so. Do you imagine all sorts of
dire consequences for acting assertive? You may have
been brought up in a household where you were taught to
"hold your tongue" and "be quiet and sit down." These
assumptions about what might happen if you are assertive
need to be examined in the clear light of day. Let's take a
look at some of them:

1. **If I'm assertive, I might upset the other person.** This is a common fear. The fact is, some people may not like it when you are assertive, but you have every right to express your feelings. Avoiding the situation only leads to a buildup of anger, a blowup, and then guilt. Or it could lead to serious interpersonal problems that could take a tremendous emotional toll (which is often converted into physical symptoms) on all involved. Either pattern can lead to binging. Still, you could be greatly overestimating the amount of emotional upset that actually would result should you confront someone. If you approach people with respect, showing sensitivity to their feelings and being honest about yours, chances of upsetting them are lessened. Just be sure you avoid belittling or putting them down. If you approach someone in a sensitive way, any upset that could occur, and it most likely won't, would be very short-lived. Of course, you must decide if you want to take the risk, but a small upset that could result may be the first step toward a real resolution of the problem. If you don't speak up, it may never be resolved. Even if the other person reacts badly, at least you know what you're up against. By remaining silent, you'll never know.

2. **If I'm assertive, the other person might try to get back at me.** There is no guarantee that this will not happen either way, just as there are no guarantees about anything in life. It would be nice if every time you were assertive the other person said, "I understand what you want and I'm going to change right away." Being assertive is really more for you and what it does to relieve pent-up feelings in you. Forget about how the other person might respond. He or she is free to choose a response just as you are. Pick your

fights. You may not wish to be assertive with a boss or teacher who does hold the power to dominate you. Ask yourself: *Does this person seem mature enough to handle an honest comment?* If the answer is no, you may choose not to be assertive. Bear in mind that this is your choice, though, and that's being assertive in itself.

3. **If I'm assertive, I might fail and look silly.** It's true that the other person may not do what you want. Even if the other person looks you in the eye and says, "No way," you still have assertive options. You can always say, "I'm sorry you feel that way. This issue is very important to me. I hope you'll think about it and decide to talk to me about it tomorrow [next week or whenever you think is appropriate]." Remember, though, the other person has a choice in the matter just as you do. Rather than look forward to the outcome, congratulate yourself on having the grace and persistence to bring the issue into the open for discussion. Bravo! You will be a better person for it.

Even if the other person tries to throw cold water on your comments and maybe even calls you overemotional or overreactive, take that and use it an assertive way, e.g., by saying, "You know what? I am emotional about this and I'm going to keep talking to you about this issue until we resolve it." This lets the other person know that you cannot be pushed around but does it in a mature and well-thought-out way.

What are some of the assertiveness situations you might encounter when you are trying to stop binging and lose weight? One might be that waiters may not bring your meal as ordered or family members may not stick to their agreement with you not to bring candy bars or potato chips into the house. If your usual response is passive (not making a fuss or even mentioning agreements) or aggressive (loud verbal conflict), then assertiveness may be helpful to you. If being assertive is something new for you, you might want to practice saying what you want to say to your bathroom mirror or record it into a tape recorder, play it back, and rerecord until it sounds exactly the way you want to sound. In psychological terms, this is called shaping, and it's a great way to make slow approximations until you have achieved the behavior you want.

The Being Assertive table here provides key aspects of being assertive:

BEING ASSERTIVE

ASSERTIVENESS ASPECT	WHAT TO DO
1. Eye contact	Look directly at the person when speaking. Eye contact is a nonverbal way of saying, *I'm sincere and firm about what I'm saying.*
2. Body posture	Stand or sit erect, an appropriate distance away, and lean in toward the other person.
3. Gestures	Emphasize important points with a gesture. Be careful of being overenthusiastic or you'll distract the other person.
4. Facial expression	Make sure your expression agrees with the words you're saying.
5. Voice	Use a well-modulated, conversational tone and emphasize important words so you'll be convincing without being intimidating.
6. Timing	Avoid hesitation and blurting things out. Ask for a few quiet moments in a private office or room. If necessary, make an appointment—even if it's with a family member or friend.

ASSERTIVENESS ASPECT	WHAT TO DO
7. Content	Be clear and direct and own your own feelings. Avoid blaiming others, arguing, or ignoring the issue. If a friend or family member keeps buying food you binge on, try saying, "I'm trying really hard not to binge. I would really appreciate it if you helped me reach my no-binging goal, so please take this ice cream out of the house and don't bring any more in."

Coping Comments Can Reduce Stress

Coping comments are a little like affirmations, but they are specifically directed at lowering your stress and they are used before, during, and after the stress situation. Here are some examples of comments to tell yourself to get through stressful times so you won't binge.

☒ Preparing for a stressor:

"What can I do to plan for stress?"
"I'm going to focus on thinking about handling this stress so I won't binge."
"I'm going to stay calm and not let stress get to me."

☒ Handling a stressor:

"I'm not going to let this upset me."
"Take a deep breath and relax."
"I don't need to binge; I'm in control of me."
"I can handle this; I'm handling it now without binge eating."
"I can focus on reading this book [exercising, drawing, watching TV] and not think 'binge.'"

☒ Rewarding yourself for handling the stressor:
"Good going. You handled that great!"
"I'm doing better every time."
"I can hardly wait to tell _____ about how I stood firm and didn't binge."
"I'm pleased with myself."

Disputing Negative Self-Talk

We all engage in almost continual self-talk while awake.
Self-talk is the internal language we use to describe and
interpret the world. When your self-talk is accurate and
realistic, you'll feel good and be healthy. When it isn't,
stress occurs. Thirty years ago Albert Ellis developed a
system to help attack irrational ideas and replace them
with more realistic interpretations and self-talk.

When you feel helpless or powerless over your binging behavior, it can help to examine your self-talk and
eliminate words and phrases that exaggerate your problems and contribute to feeling helpless. When words like
I don't have any willpower or *I've really blown it* creep
in, dispute them. Realize you don't have a character flaw
and you haven't blown anything that can't be fixed, even
if you ate half a pie or eight pieces of chocolate cake. No
one is perfect. Everyone makes mistakes. Maybe you ate
that pie or cake because you were stressed out or angry or
just hungry. Next time, you will take steps to make sure
you aren't so stressed out or angry or hungry. It's OK.
You're OK.

When you find yourself using exaggerations such as
always, awful, essential, every, horrible, terrible, and *totally,* remember that using these words—and holding the
beliefs that support the use of these words—is stressful.

A common form of negative self-talk is statements that
"awfulize" experience. Take a look at the list of negative
self-talk here and the way you can dispute these ideas if
they creep into your thinking patterns:

NEGATIVE SELF-TALK	WAYS TO DISPUTE NEGATIVE SELF-TALK
I'll never be able to stop binge eating.	I've got to start somewhere and I've decided to eat at least two of my "forbidden" foods each week, eat more fiber, and drink ten glasses of water every day. It's impor-

NEGATIVE SELF-TALK	WAYS TO DISPUTE NEGATIVE SELF-TALK
	tant to have a plan and work toward it if I want to stop binge eating.
I look terrible. I'm so fat and I'll never lose all this weight.	It doesn't help to awfulize about my weight. No one faints or laughs when I walk by because of the way I look. If I follow my plan, I'll start to lose weight and I'll feel better about myself.
I have to lose twenty pounds fast.	Losing weight quickly is stressful to my body and is apt to result in regaining it. I'm better off losing weight slowly. It took time to get into this binge-eating pattern and it's not going to disappear overnight. I just need to keep working toward my goal.
Even if I stop binge eating and lose weight, I'll just gain it back again.	I'm still learning how to manage my weight and I can expect some fluctuation in my weight. That doesn't mean I won't be successful.
It's impossible for me to stop eating doughnuts once I have one.	I have the power to resist eating doughnuts or anything else I choose to. I'm in charge of my eating habits.
I can't stand being so regimented and not being able to eat what I want when I want.	I can stand whatever I need to stand to attain my goals. It's worth it to me to follow a plan so I can stop binge eating.

Imagery Methods

Imagery is a way to use your imagination to reduce stress, remain calm, and keep from binge eating. You've probably had plenty of experience with imagery: dreams, daydreams, and fantasies are all examples of the strong images your brain can generate. Imagery provides direct access to your subconscious mind, bypassing your logical brain that leads you to worrying and to more stress. Imagery can help you cut through rumination to get to the core of what's bothering you, helping reduce your stress. Imagery is also valuable when you want to solve problems, prepare for upcoming situations, enhance healing, or decrease the influence of negative feelings and relationships. See the boxes that follow for directions on how to use imagery for each of these situations:

USING IMAGERY TO SOLVE PROBLEMS

1. Find a quiet spot and sit in a relaxed position.

2. Close your eyes.

3. Condense the problem to three to five words. (If you're having trouble doing this, picture yourself telling the problem to a friend.)

4. Ask yourself: "Am I ready to solve this problem?" Wait for an answer. If the answer is yes, proceed to Step 5. If the answer is no, choose another problem.

5. Place the problem in a frame, using a color of your choice to create a border.

6. See the solution in a frame next to the problem. Use a border of a different color.

USING IMAGERY TO PREPARE FOR AN UPCOMING SOLUTION

1. Choose a situation you are nervous about.

2. Assume a comfortable position with your body relaxed and your eyes closed.

3. Imagine yourself as the director of a movie that you start to run in your mind's eye. Remind yourself that as director, you can stop or start the movie at any point you wish. You are in control.

USING IMAGERY TO PREPARE FOR AN UPCOMING SOLUTION (CONT.)

4. Imagine everything about the situation, picturing what is said, what you feel, what the other people in the situation say and do. When you notice yourself becoming uncomfortable, stop the movie in your mind and go back to focusing on relaxing your body. When you feel relaxed again, begin the movie at the spot a little before you started to feel uncomfortable. Work back and forth between the movie in your mind and relaxing until you can complete the whole situation while remaining relaxed.

USING IMAGERY TO ENHANCE HEALING

The following universal images can be used for:

Constipation: picture a logjam breaking up or waste moving easily and freely through your intestines.

Fatigue: picture yourself filling up with energy and vitality.

Hot areas: imagine coolness, e.g., submerging the area in cool water.

Dry areas: imagine the area becoming moist, e.g., a gentle river moving over it.

Moist areas: imagine the area becoming dry, e.g., a desert growing there.

Itching or pain: imagine coolness or an ice cube in the area.

Gynecological disorders: imagine a warm pelvis.

Anger: imagine peace, love, and harmony.

Chronic sinus problems: imagine tubes opening and draining or a sink unclogging in the area.

Tense muscles: imagine the muscles getting wider and longer, unknotting and relaxing.

USING IMAGERY TO DECREASE PAINFUL OR NEGATIVE FEELINGS

1. Listen to a relaxation tape first.

2. Then picture the painful or negative feelings.

3. Picture placing the painful or negative feelings in a container of your choice.

4. Close and lock the container and send it far away where your feelings can no longer influence you.

Self-Massage

Humans need comforting touch to thrive. If you have someone to provide it for you, that's great. When that special someone is not available, try self-massage. It is very relaxing and healing. Use the directions that follow or create your own!

1. Find a quiet spot.
2. Put on some soft music.
3. Sit down in a comfortable chair.
4. Loosen any tight clothing.
5. Kick off your shoes.
6. Rub your hands together gently.
7. Place your palms over your ears for a minute or two; thank your ears for doing such a good job of hearing.
8. Place your palms over your eyes for a minute or two; thank your eyes for doing such a good job of seeing.
9. Place your palms on the top of your head for a minute or two; thank your brain for helping you think straight. Gently massage your scalp, slowly moving down the back of your head. Massage your forehead, temples, cheeks, jaw, and neck. As you massage here and the rest of

your body, if you find any tight or sore spots, linger there a little longer until it feels relaxed, tingly, and loose.

10. Massage across your shoulders, letting your worries roll across your shoulders, down your arms (as you massage them), and out your fingertips (rubbing down each finger and gently tugging it out and letting go).

11. Massage your upper back, under your arms, and down the sides of your ribs.

12. Massage down your chest and ribs. Thank your heart for beating and keeping you alive. Thank your lungs for helping you to bring in clear, fresh air.

13. Massage your waist, front and back.

14. Massage your abdomen, gently pushing in as you move down and around, covering the area down to your legs.

15. Massage your lower back and hips.

16. Move down your legs, ankles, and feet and out your toes.

17. Rest for a minute with your eyes closed and tune into your body. If there is any other area that needs more massage, provide it.

Thought Stopping

Use thought stopping when nagging thoughts keep after you to binge. Think, say, or picture the word *STOP*. Make it big, red, and bold. If that doesn't work, use a buzzer or a bell to signal yourself to stop, or wear a rubber band around your wrist and snap it when the unwanted thoughts occur. Next, say a positive, assertive statement to replace the noncontructive image behavior. Some examples follow:

- I can eat three meals a day and feel satisfied; I do not need to binge.

- I am in control of what I eat.
- I am confident in my ability to stop binging.

Time Management

Do you find yourself rushing, feeling fatigued or listless, with many slack hours of nonproductive activity, chronic missing of deadlines, insufficient time for rest or personal relationships, or a sense of being overwhelmed by demands and details? There are three steps to effective time management:

1. Establish priorities.
2. Eliminate low-priority tasks.
3. Learn to make decisions.

The first step toward managing your time more efficiently is to chart how you are spending your time. Carry a small notebook with you for three days and write down the number of minutes you engage in each activity. Divide the notebook into three sections: Waking through Lunch, After Lunch through Dinner, and After Dinner until Retiring. After three days, total the amount of time you spent doing each activity. See Claudia's Time Management Assessment for an example:

CLAUDIA'S TIME MANAGEMENT ASSESSMENT

ACTIVITY	MINUTES SPENT	ACTIVITY	MINUTES SPENT
WAKING THROUGH LUNCH:		**AFTER LUNCH THROUGH DINNER:**	
Lying in bed awake	30	Making sales calls	90
Showering	20	Daydreaming about food	35

ACTIVITY	MINUTES SPENT	ACTIVITY	MINUTES SPENT
Dressing	25	Writing reports	45
Reading a magazine	25	Socializing	20
		Driving home	30
Driving to work	30		
		Eating dinner	5
Filing	30		
		AFTER DINNER UNTIL SLEEP:	
Daydreaming	15		
Computer/ Internet	60	Watching TV	120
		Binge eating, refrigerator	50
Meeting	40		

After Claudia looked at her assessment, she made the decision to do the following:

1. Get up when the alarm rings and limit my shower to five minutes.
2. Take a late lunch so I can do more work when I'm productive and the office is quiet: 11:00 A.M. to 2:00 P.M.
3. Use thought stopping to limit daydreaming about food and binging.
4. Take a class or go out with friends in the evening so I won't binge.

Claudia's next step was to set priorities. She made a list of things she wanted to accomplish and compared it to how she spent her time. She pictured herself being told she had only three months to live and imagined how she wanted to spend the remaining time. At the top of her list was going to community college and becoming a dental assistant. She hated her job and wanted to make more money. Although she'd wanted to go back to school for years, she was overwhelmed by the idea. She decided to break her goal down into manageable steps:

1. Call the college and get a course catalog.
2. Talk with a friend who is a student there.
3. Attend orientation day at the college.
4. Register for classes.
5. Purchase books and study materials.

Claudia still felt a little overwhelmed, so she broke down these manageable steps into a daily "To Do" list that included everything she wanted to accomplish that day. She rated each item as top, middle, or low priority and worked only on the top-priority items. After a few days, she she discovered some ways to make time:

1. Always put yourself first and everything else second. If you don't, you'll be too stressed to add value to anyone's life. Nurture yourself first and you'll have plenty to give to others.
2. Stop taking care of everyone else. Instead, teach them how to take care of themselves. You build strength in others by giving them the chance to try.
3. Build a support team of experts you can call on for help. You can't do it all yourself.
4. Learn to say no to unreasonable requests. Remind yourself this is your life and your time to spend as best benefits you. If you have trouble saying no, practice on telemarketers. Tape a message to your phone and calendar or daily planner to remind yourself not to overcommit.
5. Build downtime into your schedule for unplanned events, interruptions, and unforeseen situations.

6. Keep a list of short five-minute tasks that can be done any time you are waiting or between other tasks.

7. Set aside several time periods a day to perform stress-reduction activities. If you are relaxed, you will use the rest of the time you have more efficiently.

8. Delegate some of your low-priority tasks to supervisees, secretaries, or your children, nieces or nephews, or in-laws.

9. Learn to do two fairly simple things at once: plan dinner while driving home or organize a letter or list while waiting in line for groceries. Make sure the second task is very simple so you don't overstress yourself.

10. Get up fifteen to thirty minutes earlier than usual every day and complete a high-priority task.

11. Limit television viewing to one hour a day. Use TV as a reward for completing your high-priority tasks and throw away your television remote: you'll save all the time you spend channel-surfing. Besides, watching one channel is less confusing, and if you have to get up to change the channel, you expend more calories!

12. Buy a stopwatch and use it to limit all your phone calls to ten minutes, unless it's a work-related conference call or to your boss.

13. Stop procrastinating. Don't put another piece of paper on your desk—do it or delegate it.

14. Check your e-mail only once a day and let everyone you e-mail know that you do this.

15. If you have a bell that rings every time you get an e-mail, turn it off.

16. Schedule a time to pay your bills once a month. Most companies will adjust their billing

schedule to yours. Consider making autopay contracts with your utility and mortgage companies.

17. Schedule everything. Write down every obligation you agree to on your calendar so that you control your day rather than letting it control you.

18. Schedule at least one day a week to focus on your most important activities.

19. Write at least three pages in your journal every day about whatever is on your mind. It will help you figure out what you want in life and move toward it.

20. Schedule one weekend a month to do nothing at all. Spend that time enjoying yourself and being joyful.

21. Start and end your day doing something that makes you feel good.

22. Focus on your possibilities, not your problems.

23. Develop another source of income so you can choose to leave your full-time job if you wish—for example, start your own home or Internet business that you can run evenings and weekends until you have built up a substantial source of funds.

24. Avoid telephone tag by desginating specific times to accept and return calls. When you leave a message on someone's voice mail, indicate the best time to call you back.

25. Tackle hard tasks first thing in the morning when you're fresh: the feeling of achievement can give your day momentum and a feeling of success.

26. Leave your day's schedule on voice mail.

27. Unplug your phone when you're busy or let your answering machine pick up.

28. Break each task into small and manageable pieces.
29. Exercise and eat right so you can stay physically and mentally alert; be sure to schedule in time to do both.
30. Trust that you can do it and then do it!

Procrastination—including daydreaming—is a great time robber. Use the following suggestions to help you make time-saving decisions:

1. Write down all the costs to you if you delay.
2. Ask yourself, "What are the payoffs to me for procrastinating?" ("No fear of failure," "Other people will do my work for me," "I'll get sympathy for being chronically unhappy.")
3. Intensify whatever you are doing to put off your decision until you get bored. You'll see that it's easier to just decide and move ahead with your life than to waste your time with fillers.
4. Take responsibility for the time you waste by writing down how many minutes you delayed.
5. When making unimportant decisions, flip a coin.
6. Take small steps toward your decisions; e.g., if you want to call for information, put a pen and pad by the phone with the number to call.
7. Get psyched: tell yourself how great you'll feel when you've finished the task.
8. Allow yourself to experience the reward of finishing something. Bask in your wonderfulness!

Quickie Stress Reducers
1. When feeling stressed, instead of reaching for a brownie or even when watching yourself reach for that doughnut, focus on the sensations of

your feet on the floor. How do they feel? Are they heavy or light? Are they cold or warm? How does the surface underneath you feel?

2. Count "one" as you inhale and "two" as you exhale for a period of two or three minutes. Picture yourself lying on a warm beach or above and away from stress on a cool mountaintop.

By the time you finish the exercises in this section, you will be so relaxed that your food craving will be gone. Weave one or more of these stress-reduction methods into your daily routines. For example, practice guided imagery while taking a shower or just before you turn off the light at night. Meditate or listen to a relaxation tape while lying in bed as a way to reduce stress and bring on peaceful sleep.

REFERENCES

1. Adami, G. F., G. M. Marinari, A. Bressani, S. Testa, and N. Scopinaro. 1998. Body image in binge eating disorder. *Obesity and Surgery* 8(5): 517–19.
2. French, S. A., R. W. Jeffery, N. E. Sherwood, and D. Neumark-Sztainer. 1999. Prevalence and correlates of binge eating in a nonclinical sample of women enrolled in a weight gain prevention program. *International Journal of Obesity and Related Metabolic Disorders* 23(6): 576–85.
3. Heatherton, T. F., and R. F. Baumeister. 1991. Binge eating as escape from self-awareness. *Psychological Bulletin* 110: 86–108.
4. Kinzl, J. F., C. Traweger, E. Trefalt, B. Mangweth, and W. Biebl. 1999. Binge eating disorder in females: A population-based investigation. *International Journal of Eating Disorders* 25(3): 287–92.
5. Lehman, A. K., and J. Rodin. 1989. Styles of self-nurturance and disordered eating. *Journal of Consulting and Clinical Psychology* 57: 117–22.
6. Sherwood, N. E., R. W. Jeffery, and R. R. Wing. 1999. Binge status as a predictor of weight loss treatment out-

come. *International Journal of Obesity and Metabolic Disorders* 23(5): 485–93.

7. Clark, C. C. 1996. What encourages and prevents students from engaging in wellness activities? *Wellness Newsletter* 5(6): 3–4.

CHAPTER 6

Step 5: Exercise Without Stress to Lose Weight

Tony, a fifty-year-old vice president of a computer sales company, has been told he needs to lose weight. He's never been much on exercise but golfs once or twice a month. Although he belongs to an exercise club, he doesn't go there very often, preferring to spend his time reading company reports or talking on his cellular phone to his salespeople. When he was in high school, he ran on the track team, but he broke his leg in a car accident and has no plans to return to running. He just doesn't see why he has to exercise and finds calisthenics and most sports boring. But he feels guilty about not taking better care of his health.

WHY EXERCISE MAY BE THE KEY TO PERMANENT WEIGHT LOSS FOR YOU

Did you know that only 22 percent of Americans are regularly active? It probably comes as no surprise that exercise can be the key to weight loss maintenance. Even though obesity and overweight are to some extent genetically determined, a recent study published in the *Annals of Internal Medicine* showed that inactivity, not genetics, is the best predictor of inability to lose weight,[1] and another report[2] provides strong support for the idea that exercise can promote long-term weight loss.

Physical exercise is not only useful for maintaining

weight loss. It can also yield psychological benefits to reduce stress and depression. And since we know that feeling stressed or depressed can end in binge eating, realizing the psychological benefits of exercise may be just the information you need to start your exercise program. Here's the proof: a large study of 3,403 participants found that men and women who exercised two or three times a week experienced significantly less depression, anger, cynical distrust, and stress than those who exercised less frequently or not at all. Regular exercisers also felt healthier and fitter and reported higher levels of a sense of coherence and a stronger feeling of social integration than those who exercised less frequently.[3] Their results indicate a strong association between feelings of enhanced well-being and regular physical exercise.

The good news is that your exercise may not need to be aerobic or intense for you to achieve feelings of well-being and stress reduction! In one study,[4] college students in two swimming classes, a yoga class, and a control-group lecture completed mood and personality inventories before and after class on three occasions. Both yoga and swimming participants reported greater decreases in scores on anger, confusion, tension, and depression than did the lecture-class control. Among the men, decreases in tension, fatigue, and anger after yoga were even significantly greater than those after swimming. Another study[5] also found that strenuous activity is not necessary to protect against stress, at least minor stress. Even nonstrenuous leisure-style physical activity provided a buffer against physical symptoms and anxiety associated with minor stresses. Yet another study[6] supports the idea that nonstrenuous exercise can have lasting weight management benefit. Researchers asked forty nonexercising overweight women between the ages of twenty-one and sixty to follow one of two fitness plans. Half attended forty-five-minute step aerobics classes three times a week. The other half walked, gardened, or took the stairs for a total of thirty minutes a day. All the women went on a low-fat diet. After four months both groups had lost an average of seventeen pounds. A year later, twice as many casual exercisers as classgoers were still logging thirty to forty-five minutes of physical activity most days. They were also less likely to have regained weight. There are now several hundred studies and over thirty analyses that review research summarizing the potential for exercise to reduce depression, anxiety, upgrade life quality, enhance self-esteem, improve mood states, increase resilience to stress, and improve sleep. Even with all this support for the benefits of exercise to lose weight and maintain weight loss, many people still hold exercise myths that can keep them from exercising.[7]

MYTHS ABOUT EXERCISE

You may not want to exercise because you believe the myths that surround it. So let's debunk those myths right now.

Myth 1. Exercising makes you tired. The fact is, the more physically fit you become, the more energy you have.

Myth 2. Exercising takes too much time. It only takes a few minutes a day to exercise. If you don't have thirty minutes in your schedule for an exercise break, find two fifteen-minute periods or even three ten-minute periods.

Myth 3. The older you are, the less exercise you need. Age shouldn't stop you. In fact, exercise at any age can increase your capacity to perform activities of daily living. Residents of nursing homes, age eighty and older, have benefited from exercise programs.

Myth 4. You have to be athletic to exercise. Most physical activities do not require any special athletic skills. In fact, many people who found school sports difficult have discovered that there are many activities that are easy to do and enjoy. A perfect example is walking——it requires no special talent, athletic ability, or equipment.

WHY EXERCISE?

We're sure you've seen diets advertised that tell you "guaranteed permanent weight loss—no exercise needed." The truth is that if you're fit and eat 1,000 calories, all them will get burned up and used up. When you're overweight and eat 1,000 calories, only some of them are used up and the remainder turns into fat. If you want to take weight off and keep it off, you need to train your body so that it burns all the calories you take in and stops storing them as fat. Long-term weight control requires a change in body chemistry. Exercise can help your body do this.

Exercise . . .

- **Makes you feel better.** Jogging, swimming and other aerobic activities make you feel better, possibly by increasing endorphins.[8, 9] Even non-strenuous forms of exercise such as qigong[10] and tai chi[11] affect neurotransmitters and reduce tension, depression, anger, fatigue, confusion, and anxiety.

- **Allows you to weigh more and look better** because muscle weighs more than fat. As we mentioned chapters ago, muscle is more important than weight. If you tone your body, you can weigh more and fit in smaller clothes and feel and look better. Not bad for thirty or forty minutes of your time three or four days a week. What else will do that for so little effort? Nothing that we know of. So, even if exercising does not appeal to you, try it anyway. You'll be surprised at how much better you look and feel after regular exercise. You'll also sleep better and have more energy.

- **Keeps your heart and lungs healthy.**
- **Can increase your coordination and ability to handle stressful situations.** Both of these qualities can help you avoid car accidents and other stressful encounters.
- **Will also help thin your blood and ward off clots.** This is especially important as you age.
- **Helps your tissues heal.** So, if you're planning on having surgery, be sure to exercise before you do because exercised tissues heal better. This probably has to do with the increase in oxygen that occurs when you move your body and the increased nourishment to your tissues when your blood circulates well.
- **Focuses your attention away from food.** You've probably been avoiding food, counting calories, and trying not to eat forbidden foods for years. Unlike avoiding food, a negative reaction, exercise is a positive action, something that can lead to a firmer and much more attractive body and you feeling good about your body no matter what size it is.
- **Increases body awareness,** something critical to accepting the way you are. We want you to be happy with your body and what it can do. The more you exercise in a safe way, the more your body will do for you and the prouder of it you'll be.
- **Can reduce anxiety and frustration and lead to feelings of well-being.** Even leisure activities like gardening can provide a buffering effect against physical symptoms and anxiety associated with minor stresses.[5]
- **Is also a great treatment for depression** because it stimulates your brain's production of norepinephrine, a hormone that helps keep you emotionally stable. Regular exercise also stimu-

lates production of endorphins, the "natural opiates" or "feel-good" brain substances that can give you a natural high. Serotonin is another brain chemical stimulated by exercise that can soothe and calm you.[12] Being able to create your own "feel-good" chemicals through exercise, instead of relying on store-bought drugs (caffeine, sugar, diet drugs, antidepressants, etc.) that can have bad side effects, is certainly a big plus.

- **Can also give you relief from the pressures of your life.** That's why it's so important to keep your mind on what you're doing when you're exercising, not on anything else. When you exercise that way, it can renew your spirit and rekindle your energy and enthusiasm.
- **Provides an easy way to share an activity with friends or family.**
- **Is a great way to meet new friends.**
- **Helps control your appetite.**
- **Builds your stamina.**
- **Helps you be more productive at work.**
- **Reduces your chances of getting a heart attack.**
- **Fights the effects of aging by slowing the rate at which enzymes decline.**

You may even know all this and still don't exercise. Maybe you're a little like Tony, the guy at the beginning of this chapter. He's so busy with the demands of his job that he has trouble finding time or interest to exercise. But by now, you've probably figured out that it's almost impossible to lose weight and keep it off by only changing what you eat. A combined program of wholesome food and exercise is best for losing weight and keeping healthy.

When you do start to exercise, do it the stress-free way and don't weigh yourself. Judge weight loss by the way you look and how your clothes fit. When you exercise regularly, you'll start to turn fat into muscle.

Exercise can be stressful if it's boring, competitive, or too difficult. Because of this, you may have begun exercise programs and then abandoned them, which in turn added even more stress to your life because you felt guilty about it, like Tony did. So start by taking things easy.

WHY IT'S IMPORTANT TO TAKE IT EASY WHEN YOU EXERCISE

Excessive exercise stresses your body and can take the fun out of activity. You need to see your health care practitioner before you exercise if you check one or more of the items below:

- ✓ You have a diagnosed heart condition.
- ✓ During or right after exercise, you frequently have pains or pressure in the left or midchest area, left neck, shoulder, or arm.
- ✓ You have had chest pain in the last month.
- ✓ You tend to lose consciousness or fall over due to dizziness.
- ✓ You feel extremely breathless after mild exertion.
- ✓ Your health care practitioner recommended blood pressure or heart medications.
- ✓ You have diagnosed bone or joint problems that could be made worse by physical activity.
- ✓ You have insulin-dependent diabetes or another diagnosed condition that needs special attention.
- ✓ You are middle-aged or older, have not been physically active, and plan a pretty vigorous exercise program.

Even if you've had a heart attack, exercise is good. It can help reduce your risk of having another one, increase

your chance of survival, and improve the quality of your
life. Just be sure you don't exercise too much. After hard
exercise, your body may need up to forty-eight hours to
recoup. What are the signs that you're exercising too
much or too often?

- poor coordination
- slower reaction time
- sleep problems
- irritability
- diarrhea
- fatigue
- muscle pain
- higher resting heart rate than you had before
- depression and apathy
- joint pain
- drawn face
- heavy-legged feeling

Moderate, varied exercise is the ticket. It will help you
lose weight and reduce stress, but response to exercise
can be unpredictable, which is why we take the position
that exercise should be engaged in for pure enjoyment,
energy, and vitality, rather than just for body sculpting or
fat or calorie burning. The simple act of moving the body
is helpful for boosting your mood, body image, and overall health.

Don't stress yourself with exercise. It's just not
healthy. Start by doing a little less than you think you can.
Don't push yourself. Work against that perfectonistic nature of yours that counts calories, stays away from forbidden foods, and punishes you if you eat too much or binge.
Take it easy. Everyone makes mistakes. Just start slowly.

WHAT KIND OF EXERCISE IS LEAST STRESSFUL FOR YOU?

Take a gander at the following table and check the items that appeal to you. When you're through you'll be able to choose a way of exercising that's right for your lifestyle and will be the least stressful for you.

CHOOSING EXERCISE THAT'S RIGHT FOR YOUR LIFESTYLE

It's not necessary to run a marathon or swim five miles to benefit from exercise, unless you wish to. Check the items below that appeal to you on the left side of the page, then see what exercise might be the least stressful for you.

THIS APPEALS TO ME	SO FOR EXERCISE I SHOULD . . .
___ enjoying what I'm doing and feeling relaxed	go ballroom or line dancing, garden, or walk
___ safety: I have arthritis, am pregnant, or am prone to falling	swim or practice tai chi
___ sculpting my body	lift weights (unless I have high blood pressure*), do targeted calisthenics
___ burning fat/calories	fast-walk, jog, tap-dance, or do cross-country skiing
___ being flexible	practice yoga or tai chi and other martial arts
___ increasing self-esteem	dance, practice martial arts, or lift weights

THIS APPEALS TO ME	SO FOR EXERCISE I SHOULD . . .
___ sleeping better	walk, bike, dance, or practice martial arts
___ rapid weight loss	jog, hike, do aerobics, row, do cross-country skiing, use the treadmill, climb stairs, run (hard on the joints), or jump rope (hard on the joints, plus could fall)

*Lifting weights can increase your blood pressure, especially if you don't breathe while exercising. If you have high blood pressure, check with your health care professional before starting a weight-lifting program.

Whichever exercise forms you choose, be sure to get a book or take a class on the best way to exercise using that method. You don't want to hurt yourself and you want to do it right to get the most benefit.

WHY WALKING IS A GOOD CHOICE

More than 70 million people walk for exercise. Walking at a brisk rate burns more calories than swimming, playing tennis or golf, or even doing low-impact aerobics.

One advantage of walking is that you don't need any high-tech equipment or to go to a health club. All you need are the right shoes. Be sure to buy walking shoes using the tips that follow:

- Shop for shoes later in the day when your feet are their largest size.
- Look for a brand with padded insoles, midsoles, and heel counters. Select a pair with a firm, thick sole that has good traction and is wide enough to wear comfortably with socks.

When walking, be sure to:

- Hold your head high. Picture a gold cord attached to the top of your head that pulls you up so you walk tall.
- Keep your neck and shoulders relaxed and your back flat.
- Step lightly, heel first.
- Roll your weight forward across the sole of your foot, gently pushing off with your toes.
- Keep your feet pointed straight ahead and your knees slightly bent.
- Swing the arm opposite the leg you're using.

Enjoy your walk!

CONSIDER WEIGHT LIFTING (RESISTANCE TRAINING)

If you're an average adult, you lose about six or seven pounds of muscle every ten years until you're forty-five. After this age, you lose even more—so you probably have about one-third fewer muscle cells than you had at age twenty. By the time you're seventy, your muscle cells are also smaller than those of a twenty-year-old. This is not due to aging. It happens because of disuse and sedentary living—you know, the couch potato or Internet life. Is this enough reason to consider weight lifting? Yes![14,15]

The American College of Sports Medicine thinks resistance training provides important benefits for people of all ages and abilities. They suggest the following when lifting free weights:

1. Use smooth, slow, and controlled motions.
2. Maintain good posture (doing it in front of a mirror helps).
3. Only move the body part you're exercising; the rest of you should remain still.

4. Eight to twelve repetitions is the right number. If that's too easy, it's time to add more weight.

5. Use eight to ten different weight-lifting exercises per set. (Remember: this can take as little as fifteen minutes, including warm-up time.)

6. Do three workouts a week, resting every other day to let your muscles recover. If you can't do that much, you can get about 75 percent of your maximum improvement from only two sessions a week. Even once a week will maintain you at your current level for several months. What a deal!

7. Be sure to include resistance training for your legs in your workout (unless you do aerobics); this can improve your ability to walk (maybe even run) and climb stairs and may prevent knee and hip injuries.

8. To keep building strength, you must keep increasing the weight you lift. But once you reach the level you want, e.g., your body is more defined and looks better even though you weigh the same, you can maintain that level with two repetitions of a particular exercise.

9. Remember to breathe! Holding your breath increases your blood pressure.

10. Stop if your muscles hurt. The old saying "no pain, no gain" is wrong and following it can be dangerous. Your muscles should feel fatigued during the last repetitions, but you shouldn't feel any sharp or piercing pains. If you do feel pain, stop that exercise immediately.

11. Start with one-pound weights and work up, consulting a specific weight-lifting exercise book.

12. If you need additional help, hire a personal trainer to show you the proper technique and

monitor your ability to do the exercises properly and safely.

BE SURE TO WARM UP AND COOL DOWN

If you plan to do anything more strenuous than slow walking, make sure you warm up and cool down your body. You don't want to hurt your muscles or risk an injury. Warming up is important for other reasons:

✓ Increases blood flow and oxygen to your muscles
✓ Sends out enzymes to burn fat

Warm-up #1

A. Shrug your shoulders a couple of times and try to touch your ears with your shoulders.
B. Sway left and right, bringing your right elbow down to your right hip and your left elbow down to your left hip.
C. Pretend you're throwing a baseball in slow motion.
D. Bend your knees (slightly and gently), look over your left shoulder, then look over your right shoulder.
E. Reach for the ceiling with your hands, then gently reach for the floor.
F. Pull your arms back as if they're oars and you're rowing a boat; swing your arms forward and back.
G. Make small circles with your ankles, pretending they are tied together. Now, keeping your knees together, make small circles with them. Next, do your hips, then your waist, then your chest, and finally your shoulders.

If you don't feel warmed up yet, repeat the preceding or try the next warm-up.

Warm-up #2

A. Reach your right hand over your left shoulder and reach your left hand up your back; try to clasp your hands behind your back. Try with the left hand over your right shoulder. Don't worry if you can't clasp your hands either way; just stretch easily in that direction and don't forget to breathe!

B. Stand with your feet three feet apart and fingers laced behind your back with your palms up. Slowly lift your arms up and over your head while lowering your head gently toward the floor. This will warm up your upper back and legs.

C. With your legs wide apart and palms on the floor, shift your hips to the left, bending the left knee, then shift your weight to the right, bending your right knee. Use a slow, controlled motion and don't worry about how far you bend your knees. This will warm up your lower body.

D. Sit on the floor with the soles of your feet together. Press your hands on the inside of your knees and hold for thirty seconds, then relax. This will warm up your hips and legs.

E. Stand about a foot away from a door. Keeping your body straight, lean against the door, bending first the right knee (feel the pull up the back of your left leg) and then the left knee.

If you would like to learn about more involved stretches, yoga is also an excellent warm-up and cooldown. Find a yoga class and join it. Not only will it keep your muscles and bones safe from injury, but it will lift your mood, too.

AVOID INJURIES

The most powerful treatment for injury is prevention. Be sure to follow the following tips:

1. **Build up your level of activity gradually over the upcoming weeks.** Don't set your goals too high at first. This way you won't be tempted to push too hard.

2. **Listen to your body.** You body will warn you with pain, light-headedness, or fatigue when you're overdoing. Pay attention to those messages and stop before you injure yourself.

3. **Pay attention to the weather conditions.** If you're exercising outside in the cold, wear warm clothes in layers that you can take off and wrap around your waist as you warm up. Wear mittens, gloves, or socks on your hands to protect them. Always wear a hat, since up to 40 percent of your body's heat can be lost through your neck and head. In hot climates, drink lots of fluids. Wear a plastic water bottle strapped to your waist if it's especially hot and wear light, loose-fitting clothes. Avoid wearing rubberized or plastic suits, sweatshirts, and sweatpants to try to lose weight; this type of clothing can cause dangerously high body temperature and result in heat stroke.

WHAT ARE THE EFFECTS OF EXERCISE ON CELLULITE?

If you have cellulite, you may be especially interested in exercise. First, let's talk about what cellulite is. Cellulite is fat that is covered by skin and support tissue that tend to pucker and wrinkle. Full-blown cellulite occurs when your connective tissue is overcome by fat accumulation.[16] Although there are no research studies on the effects of exercise on these fat deposits, observation of clients who begin weight-lifting and regularly doing leg lifts reveals reduced cellulite. It makes logical sense: if fat is replaced with muscle through exercise, there will be less fat accumulation and therefore less cellulite.

HOW OFTEN AND FOR HOW LONG SHOULD YOU EXERCISE?

Since exercise may be critical to controlling your weight, try to exercise every single day. That may sound like a lot now, but soon it will become part of your daily regime, just like brushing your teeth or going to sleep.

Make sure to keep your exercise at a low-enough level so that you can exercise for about thirty minutes each day. If you're doing aerobics, that may be too much to start. If it is, then try fifteen minutes twice a day. Get an aerobics tape or tape aerobics shows on your TV and replay them. But remember—don't tire yourself out or stress yourself. Easy does it! If you try to do too much, you will become frustrated and may give up on exercise. Plan your exercise so that you don't overdo. Here's how one of our clients worked this out:

> Rhonda weighed 300 pounds when she decided to start exercising. She couldn't walk farther than down her driveway when she started. So, she walked down her driveway and back in the morning and took the same trip in the afternoon and again after dinner. As the weight began to come off, Rhonda slowly increased her walk from her driveway, to the end of the block, to two blocks, to a mile. Now, at 180 pounds, she is walking two miles a day. She said that if she had to walk two miles when she first started, she would have quit. By starting slowly and working up to her exercise goal, she felt good about herself and her new body. You can do it, too!

OVERCOMING YOUR OBSTACLES TO EXERCISING

We know that your best intentions to exercise don't always translate into action. It's so much easier to just sit in a chair and read or get dressed and have a cup of coffee than it is to slip an aerobics video in your VCR and trot around or go outside for a walk before work. It's just human nature sometimes to take the line of least resistance. But if you want to lose fat, exercise it must be. Learn how to dispute your exercise excuses. See the following table for some ideas:

DISPUTING YOUR EXERCISE EXCUSES

EXCUSE	DISPUTE
I'm too busy.	What's more important than my body? I need to keep exercise a high priority in my life. It takes time, but I'm worth it!
I can't motivate myself.	Sure I can. I just have to start doing it. Once I get going and I see and feel results, it will get easier and easier.
Other things are more important.	Taking care of myself is as important as anything else. I'll be able to do other things more efficiently after I exercise, and I'll be healthier, too! I can put my mind on cruise control while I exercise and think about the other important things I need to think about later.
I don't feel good.	Unless I have a fever or am staying-in-bed sick, exercise is good for me. I don't need to break any records and can do less, but I'll feel better after I exercise—I always do. Even a reduced exercise session is better than nothing, so here I go!
I'd rather watch TV.	But watching TV is a waste of time. I'm committed to improving my health and looking better, and exercise is the ticket!

EXCUSE	DISPUTE
I'm worn out.	Exercise will energize me, so I need to exercise even more now. My fatigue is mental fatigue, and a physical workout is just what I need.
I didn't get enough sleep.	I can rest later. For now, exercise is important, and it will help me to sleep later on. I must remember that exercise will energize me.
I'll exercise later or maybe tomorrow.	Now is the time I've set aside to exercise, and I'm going to do it now. I'll be so proud of myself for doing it, and I'll feel really good, too.
OK, so I missed one exercise session. Big deal.	It is a big deal if I miss my exercise session. I promised myself I'd exercise and my commitment to me is the most important commitment I can make. If I can't trust myself, who can I trust?

Still need some motivation? Here are some tips for starting and sticking with an exercise program:

- **Wait for two hours after a meal to exercise.** Let your body digest the food you've eaten, then exercise.
- **When running, walking, or skiing, search out smooth surfaces.** Soft, even surfaces are safer and better for your joints and feet.
- **When exercising outside, wear brightly colored clothes and reflectors at night.** It's safer.
- **Start small.** Don't think you can jog two miles your first time out. Walk half a block instead. If you are significantly overweight and over thirty years old, check in with your health care

provider before you start exercising. Caution is always best.

- **Make it fun.** Pretend you're an Olympic race-walker and put a banner across your chest or go bicycling with your grandchild or a neighborhood kid. Do whatever you have to do to make exercising fun.
- **Use proper equipment and clothing when exercising.**
- **Vary the way you exercise to counter boredom.** Walk one day; use weights the next; swim the next. Include at least ten minutes of warm-up and cooldown exercises in your exercise program to avoid injury.
- **Find ways to work exercise into your daily routine.** Park a few blocks away from work or your next appointment. Walk or dance during your lunch break. Walk upstairs instead of taking the elevator. Do housework at a brisker pace. Mow your own lawn. Carry your own groceries. Choose an activity, like dancing, rather than going to see a movie or reading a book. Take activity breaks rather than coffee or food breaks throughout the day.
- **Focus on the positives of exercising.** Keep an ongoing record of your moods and compare the differences in your moods, energy, relaxation, concentration, bowel habits, and sleep patterns when you exercise regularly.
- **Use imagery to encourage yourself.** Whenever you find it difficult to get yourself out of bed or off the couch, picture yourself toned, radiant, energetic, and healthy after exercising.
- **Work with a supportive peer or trainer or join an exercise club.** Spend more time with people who are devoted to fitness and health. If you have difficulty getting yourself motivated,

join an exercise club or hire a personal trainer. It will be worth it! The support and enthusiasm will rub off on you. Spend less time with couch potatoes and naysayers who tease you about exercising. If they harass you, tell them to join in the fun or leave you alone.

- **Walk after every meal, even if it's only for five minutes.** It will mark a definite end to eating or snacking and signify that it's time for another activity; plus your metabolism has to work harder and burn more calories. Research shows that not only does your body burn more calories after an exercise session, but also your metabolism stays elevated for hours after each time you exercise.

- **Schedule your exercise sessions and put them on your calendar.** Block out that half hour or hour so nothing can interfere with exercise time.

- **Focus on time spent on the activity, not distance or being energetic.** Research shows you'll be more consistent in exercising if you focus on time, not distance. Even if you feel sluggish or tired, just put in your time. Then, when you feel really great, go all out and enjoy the feeling of your body moving gracefully through space.

- **Reward yourself for meeting your exercise goals.** After a month of exercising, treat yourself to a meal out or a new pair of shoes.

- **Remind yourself of your successes.** Exercise will bring its own rewards, but it's important that you also remind yourself of the great work you're doing. Post your exercise goals, mottos, pictures of your ideal self, affirmations, and words of encouragement around you. Show you that you like what you're doing!

CHOOSING AN EXERCISE GOAL THAT'S RIGHT FOR YOU

Now that you have enough information to choose well, it's time to pick an exercise goal that's right for you. Here are some goals to choose from. Select one of these and make an agreement with yourself to follow through, or devise your own exercise goal. It's all up to you.

___ I promise myself I will walk twenty minutes a day starting tomorrow.

___ I promise myself I will go dancing for at least an hour three times every week.

___ I promise myself I will work in my garden for an hour four days a week.

___ I promise myself I will buy a weight-lifting book and follow the instructions.

___ I promise myself I will sign up for a tai chi class and participate in every class.

___ I promise myself I will turn on the television before work and actively participate in one of the exercise programs.

___ I promise myself I will buy a treadmill or stair climber and use it three times a week for twenty minutes.

___ I promise myself I will join a health club and go there and actively exercise at least three times every week.

___ I promise myself I will: _____

REFERENCES

1. Samarus, K. 1999. Genetic and environmental influences on total-body and central abdominal fat: The effect of physical activity in female twins. *Annals of Internal Medicine* 130: 873–82.

2. Sarlio-Lahteenkorva, S., and A. Rissanen. 1998. Weight loss maintenance: Determinants of long-term success. *Eating and Weight Disorders* 3(3): 131–35.

3. Bryne, A., and D. F. Byrne. 1993. The effect of exercise on depression, anxiety and other mood states: A review. *Journal of Psychosomatic Research* 37: 565–74.

4. Berger, B. G., and D. R. Owen. 1992. Mood alteration with yoga and swimming: Aerobic exercise may not be necessary. *Perceptual Motor Skills* 75(3): 1331–43.

5. Carmack, C. L., E. Boudreaus, M. Amaral-Melendez, P. J. Brantley, and C. de Moor. 1999. Aerobic fitness and leisure physical activity as moderators of the stress-illness relation. *Annals of Behavioral Medicine* 21(3): 251–57.

6. Andersen, R. E., T. A. Wadden, S. J. Bartlett, B. Zemel, T. J. Verde, and S. C. Franckowiak. 1999. Effects of lifestyle activity vs. structured aerobic exercise in obese women: A randomized trial. *Journal of the American Medical Association* 281(4): 335–40.

7. Fox, K. R. 1999. The influence of physical activity on mental well-being. *Public Health Nutrition* 2(3A): 411–18.

8. Kraemer, R. R., E. O. Acevedo, D. Dzelwaltowski, J. L. Kilgore, G. R. Kraemer, and V. D. Castracane. 1996. *International Journal of Sports Medicine* 17(1): 12–16.

9. Dey, S. 1994. Physical exercise as a novel antidepressant agent: Possible role of serotonin receptor subtypes. *Physiology and Behavior* 55(2): 323–29.

10. Liu, B., J. Jiao, and Y. Li. 1990. Effect of qigong exercise on the blood level of monoamine neurotransmitters in patients with chronic disease. *Chung Hsi I Chieh Ho Tsa Chih* 10(4): 205.

11. Jin, P. 1989. Changes in heart rate, noradrenaline, cortisol and mood during tai chi. *Journal of Psychosomatic Research* 33(2): 107–206.

12. Hassmen, P., N. Koivula, and A. Uutela. 2000. Physical exercise and psychological well-being: A population study in Finland. *Preventive Medicine* 30(1): 17–25.

13. Wang, H. Y., T. R. Gashore, and E. Friedman. 1995. Exercise reduces age dependent decrease in platelet protein kinase C activity and translocation. *Journal of Gerontology and Biological Science and Medicine* 50A(1): M12–M16.

14. Campbell, W. W., M. C. Crim, V. R. Young, and W. J. Evans. 1994. Increased energy requirements and changes in body composition with resistance training in older

     adults. *American Journal of Clinical Nutrition* 60(2): 167–75.

15. Ryan, A. S., R. E. Pratley, D. Elahi, and A. P. Goldberg. 1995. Resistive training increases fat-free mass and maintains RMR despite weight loss in postmenopausal women. *Journal of Applied Physiology* 79(3): 818–23.

16. Pierard, G. E., J. Nizet, and C. Pierard-Franchimont. 2000. Cellulite: From standing fat herniation to hyperdermal stretch marks. *American Journal of Dermatopathology* 22(1): 34–7.

CHAPTER 7

Step 6: Subdue Other Life Stressors That Keep You from Losing Weight

Resentment and unresolved anger can quickly turn to overeating and binge eating to "stuff the feelings in." Sometimes, such negative patterns can be found in relationships with your loved ones. Changing these negative patterns can play an important, even essential, role in weight loss. Just as research shows that having a supportive other person can be a great help in losing weight, it's possible to be locked in destructive relationships that can stop you from losing weight. Take a look at the case study that follows. It shows how a family can be nonsupportive, preventing successful weight loss.

Kathleen, age forty-two, was the mother of four teenage children. She worked as a middle school teacher and frequently tutored students after school to make extra money. Her husband demanded a hot meal every evening, including meat and potatoes and dessert, and chided her when she tried to eat vegetables and rice or skip dessert. At other times, he complained about her weight but then brought home boxes of candy and pies from the local bakery. Her two sons and two daughters came and went from the dinner table, each wanting something different to eat.

Feeling guilty about being away from home so much, she tried to cook whatever each wanted but felt completely frustrated that no one seemed to appreciate her efforts.

Kathleen's story is an example of how guilt, stress, and lack of support from her family helped keep her locked in an overweight situation she detested. Take a look at the following form and see which, if any, of your relationships may be toxic, hindering your weight loss:

COULD YOUR RELATIONSHIPS BE HINDERING YOUR WEIGHT LOSS?

Circle YES or NO in answer to the questions below to find out how your relationships with other people may be interfering with your ability to weigh what you want to weigh. The more YES answers you've circled, the more relationship stress is hindering your weight loss.

1. My spouse/boyfriend/girlfriend is not supportive of my efforts to lose weight. YES NO

2. My family teases and/or scolds me about my weight. YES NO

3. My friends tease and/or scold me about my weight. YES NO

4. My children tease and/or scold me about my weight. YES NO

5. I am resentful of at least one past or current relationship. YES NO

6. I have at least one person I must deal with at work who is difficult. YES NO

7. At least one person in my life does not treat me with respect. YES NO

8. I feel that at least one person in my life does not hear me when I try to tell him/her something. YES NO

GETTING THE IMPORTANT PEOPLE IN YOUR LIFE TO SUPPORT YOUR WEIGHT LOSS PLANS

No matter how hard you try to lose weight, it won't work if the important people in your life sabotage you. What words can you say to family, friends, or coworkers to obtain their support in losing weight? Let's take a look at some statements you could use to gain their support:

- "I'm trying to lose weight and I could really use your help. Would you be willing to help me by not bringing home potato chips and ice cream?"
- "I need praise when I meet my goal and silence about my setbacks. Nagging is never helpful, so please don't nag me."
- "I get angry when I'm teased. Please support me during this time when I'm trying to lose weight."
- "Instead of teasing me, what about helping me by going for walks with me or eating healthy food when you're with me?"

Here are some other great ways to get your partner, family, or friends to be more supportive of your efforts to lose weight:

1. **Cook a healthy meal for the family and ask for comments and their support.** Tell everyone at the table that you are trying to lose weight and you need their support introducing healthier foods into your eating plan. Ask other family members to volunteer to cook a healthy meal one of the next evenings.
2. **Call a partner, family, and friends meeting and ask each person for support.** Partner, family, and friends meetings are a good way to work out difficulties with other people in your life. Settle on a day and time when everyone's usually around or can be around and set a meeting for

that time. At first people may grumble, make excuses, and not want to show up, but be persistent. Tell them they can get something out of the meeting, too. Ask them to write down one thing they'd like to change about how things operate when you're together and bring it to the meeting. Assure them that it will be brought up for discussion and that you will support their right to find a solution if they will help you introduce healthy eating patterns and supportive interactions. On the day of the meeting, gather everyone together and ask each person to fold up the piece of paper with the one thing he or she would like to see changed in the group written on it and hand it to you. Add your wish to introduce healthy eating patterns and supportive interactions. Draw one piece of paper and read that person's wish aloud. Allow ten to fifteen minutes per person for a discussion of that person's wish. Tell the group that everyone can have his or her say, but no arguing or making fun of anyone's comments. As soon as a plan for the first person's wish has been agreed upon, choose another piece of paper out of the hat or bowl and continue. If you encounter difficulties facilitating a family meeting, you might want to take an assertiveness class to help raise your level of assertiveness.

Couple/Family/Friends Closeness Exercise

Try this Couple/Family/Friends Closeness Exercise at your next meeting or gathering to enhance positive feelings and support. Tape the instructions on a tape recorder and play it back for the whole group to follow.

Instructions:

1. Gather in a circle and stand without touching one another.

2. Let your arms hang loosely and comfortably by your sides.

3. Close your eyes and gently breathe in, letting the breath go to your abdomen, your center.

4. Breathe in again and send a wave of relaxation through your body, exhaling and picturing the breath going out through your fingertips.

5. Continue to breathe in and out. Imagine you are a tree, with roots growing out through your toes and fingertips, providing you with a solid base of support.

6. Take in strength and flexibility through the earth below you, helping you grow.

7. The next time you breathe in, breathe in safety and security and love. Let go of all resentment, anger, and conflict as you exhale. Feel yourself relaxing.

8. Join hands with the people on each side of you.

9. On your next inhalation, send a wave of energy and love to everyone in the circle. Feel their love and strength returning to you. (Pause five seconds.)

10. Continue to inhale and exhale, experiencing how good it feels to give and receive love. (Pause thirty seconds.)

11. Gently squeeze the hands you are holding, then let go, taking their love and strength with you.

12. Slowly open your eyes.

13. (Optional) Move forward and join in a group hug.

CHOOSE A ROLE MODEL FOR SUPPORT

Let's say you can't find a supportive person among your family or friends who agrees to help you lose weight or at least not nag you or sabotage your efforts. What then?

You might choose a role model, someone who repre-

sents what you want to be. It can be a real-life person or a
fantasy person.

Take a minute to decide who that person might be and
write his or her name here: _____.

OK, now that you know who your role model is, write
down what qualities that person has that you would like
to have: _____

_____.

Imagine that person as clearly as you can in your
mind's eye. Enlarge that image, taking careful notice of
all the details. Freeze-frame the detailed image and put it
somewhere inside you where it will always be available.

Now you have someone who can provide you with
support, someone who will never nag or sabotage, and
someone who is always available. You have someone you
created and can change any time you want to into a more
supportive, encouraging helper.

What else could you want?

CONFLICT CAN KEEP YOU FROM LOSING WEIGHT

Not all relationship conflicts can be resolved in the ways
suggested previously. Sometimes, more advanced conflict management techniques may be needed. Conflict
can keep you from losing weight if you are using a lot of
your energy to resolve it. Conflict includes many behaviors, from quiet arguing, to quarreling, to outright physical aggression. Verbal conflict is a natural occurrence in
any relationship, but if this conflict is excessive or if you
are in a relationship with physical violence present, seek
help from a counselor and/or the police.

It's healthy to have a little verbal conflict in a relationship, because if there wasn't any, that would be a sign that
someone is too submissive or may be stockpiling hurts.
Take a moment and think about if there is positive conflict in your relationships or you are submissive and
could be stockpiling resentment. Whether your conflict
arises from issues of power, use of resources, needs, or

differing value systems, the end result is increased stress. The good news is that conflict can be resolved and that it can be healthy if it promotes open communication. If you ignore conflict it's very likely to go underground, but it comes out in a new disguise from time to time, sometimes as binge eating.

You can get into a conflict situation if you assume other people see things the way you do. A lot of the time, that simply isn't true. For example, you may be a very private, quiet, laid back, trusting, warm, sympathetic, nonconfrontational type of person who prefers to make small talk or listen. When others tell you to stop being overly emotional or irrational, you may feel victimized and shut down and close the other person out so you don't lose control of yourself, become hysterical, or turn your anger inward and get depressed.

You may assume everyone else is like that, too. But there are people who do not decide things based on their feelings; they're more concerned with facts. They want to control situations; they're enthusiastic, animated, manipulative, decisive, and confrontational. If you appeal to their feelings, you will get nowhere. They want only the facts but aren't above changing the topic of the discussion to one that puts them in a good light. Such people always want the last word, will sulk if they don't get what they want, and will hit back hard if you confront them about it.

Then there are the people who analyze everything. They are serious and sensible, methodical, and self-controlled. They pride themselves on being emotionally uninvolved. If you confront them about their lack of feeling, they may hit back hard, too, attacking any weakness in your reasoning, lose patience, turn off, try to regain control over the situation, or get depressed.

And there are even people who have great charm and style and appear to be somewhat aloof and removed from relationships but try to establish a superior position in relation to you. They rarely display extremes of behavior or emotion; you won't hear them raising their voice or disagreeing violently. But they are often depressed and self-involved. When you call them on their behavior, they may boil over into anger, become more depressed, or cut you off.

In which of these portraits do you most see yourself? In which do you see those around you?

It's important that you know your style and which communication style the other important people in your life have. Once you know that, you can start to resolve any conflicts you have with them.

One way to read styles is to pay close attention to nonverbal communication. This may take some practice, although you have probably been unconsciously reading and responding to other people's nonverbal communication for years. Bringing this information into conscious awareness will provide you with even more clues about how to reduce conflict. When eye, mouth, and body movement conflict with what is being said, pay attention to the gestures. They are probably more in tune with what is really meant. The face is probably the easiest part of the body to read because the muscles of the face react to stress and are easily viewed. Keep in mind the person's "normal" look and watch for eyebrow, forehead, lip, and tongue changes. Also, watch for tics or spasms. Be aware of changes in skin tone. Reddening or paling can communicate a mood shift. Train yourself to pick up eye changes; they can betray emotions that are not being shared in words.

RESOLVING CONFLICT

Once you know what is behind the conflict, you can begin to make a plan to resolve it. What are some ways to resolve conflict? One way to do this is to be willing to listen actively to each other and address underlying issues. Good negotiation skills are necessary in this process. All relationships are a study in negotiation. To get along with another person, you must be willing to give and take. Many people don't have those skills. If you don't, you might consider taking an assertiveness course.

"Claiming" is an important part of conflict resolution. Claiming includes verbally owning your feelings when you are upset, by a statement such as: "I feel angry when you tease me." This sentence clearly claims the emotion as yours and allows the other person to respond to a clear message.

Blaming messages communicate that the other person in the relationship is responsible for your feelings. For example, a blaming statement might be: "You make me so angry when you tease me." The result of a blaming statement is usually a defensive response from the other person. Blaming statements can be turned into jointly owned issues with comments such as, "As a family, we don't talk honestly with one another," or, "As a couple, we don't take much time to have fun together," or, "Our family doesn't show much affection and I wish we did."

Quarrels are not a good conflict resolution tactic. During quarrels, there is an attack on the other person's values. Insults and personal attacks are often hurled in the heat of a quarrel. The result can be many bad feelings. To prevent quarrels, try to:

- Identify the times when quarrels are most likely to occur and avoid discussions at those times.
- Notice the danger signals that lead up to a quarrel and refuse to engage in a quarrel.
- Identify what triggers quarrels for you and use stress management procedures (see chapter 5) to reduce them.
- Agree on a "no fight" signal when everyone involved must become quiet and calm. A common signal is the time-out sign (making a *T* with your two index fingers). No words are used; just make the sign with your fingers and repeat it

until the other person stops trying to badger you. If the sign alone doesn't work, say, "Time out. We'll talk later," and leave the area until you've cooled down.[1]

It will also help to defuse conflict if you reinforce people's own self-image. Communication experts D. G. Foster and M. Marshall suggest these ways to get through to others in their book *How Can I Get Through to You*[2]:

- To people who focus mostly on feelings, you might say, using as much warmth as you can muster, "I like that you're always so thoughtful and try hard not to hurt other people's feelings and never try to dominate or make a decision without carefully considering every aspect of the situation."
- To people who are really hardworking, you might say, very wholeheartedly, "I like that you get so passionate and enthusiastic about everything, that you always deal with things quickly and efficiently, that you're such a hard worker, and that you're never a follower, always a leader."
- To people who are so self-controlled, you can say, "I like that you're always so coolheaded in a crisis, that you always fight for what you believe in, that you're systematic and focused, and that you can make sense out of the most difficult information."
- To people who try to be superior, you can say respectfully, "I like that you make things happen when we can't, that you're so exciting to be around, that you get to the heart of everything, and that you have so much charisma."

Once the important people in your life feel understood, you'll be surprised how much easier it is to talk to them.

SOLVING PROBLEMS THAT LEAD TO STRESS

You probably have some stresses in your life that require action and problem-solving. If you don't already have problem-solving skills, this section may reduce a lot of stress for you. You can learn to cope with everyday problems by becoming aware of what is causing you stress and evaluating different courses of action to reduce that stress.

Like so many things in life, problem solving requires a "take charge" attitude. You may do just fine "taking charge" at work or school but have difficulty doing the same thing in your personal life. There you may feel inhibited and insecure and fall into old family patterns. That's pretty normal. But did you know that you can overcome that?

You can. You may feel down or frustrated, but it's still possible to be in charge of your emotions. How do you do that?

It's not that difficult if you know the steps to follow. They are listed here with examples of how to use them. We have confidence you can do this!

1. **Define the problem.** Make sure you do this in very precise terms. Problems can seem overwhelming when they're vague. For example, saying, "I hate my job, so I overeat," is general; so is, "My family expects too much and that causes me to overeat." You have to define what you hate about your job or what your family expects more specifically if you want to come up with a solution. Ask yourself, "What exactly do I hate about my job?" Get specific about the exact things you hate. Specific problem statements might be: "I hate that I have to do everyone else's work and when I get behind I overeat," or, "I hate that when I have to call customers I get nervous and eat too many snacks." The same

holds for the vague statement about your family expecting too much. Ask yourself, "What exactly does my family expect me to do?" The difference between a specific statement and a vague one is when the problem is stated specifically, it almost leads you to what you have to do to find a solution.

2. **Brainstorm a solution.** The next step in problem solving is finding a solution. Ask yourself, "What has to happen so that this problem is no longer a problem?" Begin to think about possible solutions. Rule out none of them yet. That's what brainstorming is all about—just letting the ideas flow. Don't worry if they make sense; just write them down as they come to mind. Don't worry if some of them sound silly or fantastic. Once you have them all written down, then is the time to decide which ones will work. Rate them from 1 (could work) to 4 (no way). Once you've rated them, focus on the number 1s. Decide which one has the very best chance of being successful. Remember, no solution is 100 percent surefire. Even if you have a little doubt about your first choice, it may be the best shot you have at solving the problem.

3. **Take action.** Now you have the problem defined and a realistic solution in hand. Maybe you'll decide to ask a coworker to switch tasks with you; everyone has parts of their jobs they hate. Hopefully, you dislike aspects that others don't, and vice versa. If your problem is that your family expects too much of you, you might ask them to share household tasks with you so you're not overwehelmed.

You might want to practice what you're going to say to your coworkers or family before speaking to them. A good way to do this is to record your voice saying what you want to say and then rate yourself on how convincing you were. If you think you weren't very convincing, keep practicing until you sound just right. If you don't have a tape recorder, you might be able to borrow one from a friend or the local library, or just go in the bathroom, shut the door, and practice talking to your mirror. This method has one advantage over the tape—you can also evaluate how you look when you speak and practice until your facial expression and gestures fit your words.

Keep in mind that problems that have been around for a while may be not be fixed in one short discussion. What you may have to do is lay the groundwork in your initial discussion with coworkers or family and then ask for their help in working out the problem. Often others do not know how you are feeling unless you tell them. After all, they're not mind readers. So, when your emotions are strong, think of an assertive way to own your feelings and discuss the issue with whoever is involved.

DEALING WITH CRITICISM

Criticism from others is very stressful and often leads to overeating. Though criticism can eat at you and make you feel bad about yourself, stay hopeful—there are ways to deal effectively with criticism[3]:

1. **Acknowledging criticism.** Just acknowledging criticism often is all that is needed. What acknowledging does is focus your energy on a positive action or clear communication. That can reduce stress and lets other people know that you heard their message and are willing to discuss it. This is important because many

times in a conversation the other person has no idea how what is said is affecting you. Some ways to acknowledge criticism are to say, "You're right; I did overeat tonight," or, "Yes, I didn't do the dishes." Both statements are assertive replies to criticism. Excuses and apologies aren't. When you were little, parents and teachers might have demanded them, but now you're an adult and you have the right to choose whether to give an explanation or not. Sometimes it's not helpful to give an explanation because that provides more ammunition for the other person to blast you with. It also doesn't present a picture of competence and being in charge of yourself. You may *choose* to give an explanation when someone criticizes you, but you don't have to. Remember, you are not obligated to explain yourself. It's all up to you.

2. **Clouding.** Clouding is a way to deal with criticism you don't agree with. It can allow you to stand your ground while still communicating with the other person. To use clouding effectively, you have to listen carefully. The idea is to agree with the part of the statement that you agree with but not agree to change. For example, if someone criticizes you for "making excuses for not working overtime" and asks, "What's the matter with you?" you could use clouding and say, "Yes, I do have many family responsibilities," or, "You're right; I guess it does seem like I give excuses." If someone criticizes your weight by saying, "Are you gaining weight?" you could say, "It may be that I've gained a few pounds."

3. **Assertive probing.** When criticism is used to avoid important feelings or desires, assertive

probing can help you to determine whether the criticism is constructive or manipulative. The aim of assertive probing is to clarify unclear comments. The first step in assertive probing is to listen carefully and find the part of the criticism most bothersome to the critic. Then ask, "What is it that bothers you about that?" For example, if your boss says, "You're not doing a very good job here," you can ask, "What is it about my work that bothers you?" As the critic explains the problem, keep asking, "What is it about that that bothers you?" When you have your answer, say, "Thanks for explaining the situation to me," and walk away. Now you have the information you need to solve the problem. (See "Solving Problems That Lead to Stress.")

4. **Broken record.** This approach is useful when other people don't seem to hear or accept what you say. You simply say it again and again . . . and again, until you're heard. Be sure to formulate a short, specific statement that tells the other person the limits of what you'll do, e.g., "I hear you saying you're upset, but I don't want to work any more overtime," or, "No, I don't want to switch schedules with you," or, "No, I can't come home for the weekend." Then, just keep saying it until the other person gives up.

5. **Content-to-process shift.** When the focus or point of the conversation drifts away from the original topic, the content-to-process shift can help you switch from what is being discussed to what is happening between you and the other person. Some comments to make are, "We're off the point; let's get back to what we were talking about," "Let's not get into a battle

about this," and even, "You seem upset. What's bothering you?"

6. **Momentary delay.** In many situations there is an implied command from the other person that a question that's been asked must be answered right away. Rather than being swayed by the emotion of the moment, take a deep breath and think about your answer. There is no question that must be answered immediately unless it is a matter of life and death. Otherwise, just say, "Give me a minute to think about this." Take your time. If you can't come up with a good answer, try approach 7.

7. **Time-out.** When the conversation reaches an impasse, suggest a time-out. During that time, use the other problem-solving steps to come up with some new responses. This approach will only work if you set a specific time to get together to work the problem out. You might say something like, "Let's sleep on this and get together tomorrow for lunch to work this out," or, "I need a day or two to think about what you said and I suggest we get together on Tuesday to discuss it."

8. **Deflection and humor.** This is a useful approach when you need to deflect or redirect an attack. The element of surprise, through either deflection or humor, can disrupt an attack. Try changing the subject ("Is that a new suit you're wearing?") or an absurd explanation ("I would have finished the report, but aliens attacked my office."). This response also helps you to take the criticism less seriously, thereby freeing you from stress. Be careful when using this technique with bosses, especially those without a good sense of humor.

9. **Joining the attacker.** When you choose to

join the attacker, you agree with the other person's right to feel as he or she does. When you join with the attacker, you take an Aiki approach, flowing with or being the water, not the rock. A sample dialogue of this technique follows:

OTHER PERSON: "I'm going to have to take some action on this."

YOU: "I dont blame you."

OTHER PERSON: "What are talking about, you don't blame me?

YOU: "It's not up to me to blame anybody. I can see you're not happy, and I can't argue with that."

OTHER PERSON: "You think you did right?"

YOU: "I guess not; you're not happy. My job is to work with you."

OTHER PERSON: "What are you talking about?"

YOU: "Let's see if we can't work something out that we can both live with. What are some of your complaints?"

10. **Parley.** This approach is most effective when you are involved in a no-win situation in which the other person is trying to make your relationship into a contest. In this case, your best response is to parley. Some comments to use are: "Let's try to work out a compromise," "Let's see if we can iron out the problem," and "If we work together, maybe we can solve both our problems."

11. **Fighting back.** This is the best response when there is no other option, it is a question of life or death, or the problem has a high priority. Fighting back means you express your anger directly and stand up to insults. Before taking

any action, ask yourself the following questions:

- Does this person have nothing to lose by being aggressive? If the answer is yes, you may want to reconsider, because the other person in the interchange may not be too reasonable.
- What is the minimum amount of energy I need in this situation to make my point?
- What is the best time and place for a confrontation?
- What is the best way to stop an attacker's advance?
- What is the best way to focus on the problem and not bring in personalities and generalities?
- What do I want my face and body to say and how can I be sure they say it?
- What spatial relationship to the other person is apt to end in harmony and how can I attain it?

Once you have your answers, devise your "fighting back" statement. You may want to create your own comment or use one of these: "I'm angry about what you said and I'd like to talk about it," or, "I feel insulted. Please don't talk to me like that. I deserve respect."

12. **Multiple attack.** When you are attacked by several people at once, it can feel quite intimidating. It you look at the geometry of the attack, you will see that for the attack to be sustained, the attackers require one another to continue the attack. Their forces create a balance when their energy is focused directly

on you. Try to keep one of your attackers between you and the others, and the attack will be defused. For example, ask that person what he or she sees as the main problem and what the rest of the people there think. When family members or peers attack, it may be best to get all the attackers together. Resist becoming defensive and be sure to practice deep breathing and relaxation to keep yourself calm. Ask each person to state his or her complaints clearly, and focus on your breathing while you listen.

ASSERT YOUR RIGHTS

As a child, you may have learned that your feelings aren't important, that you must respect people in authority, and that you have to accommodate others and help people in need. You may even have been taught that it's selfish to put your needs first or that it's shameful to make mistakes. Now, you're grown-up and you have rights. Claim your personal rights in all your relationships.

You have the right to:

- be treated with respect
- follow your own values and guidelines as long as you don't interfere with the rights of others
- have feelings
- live by your own opinions and convictions
- change your mind
- make mistakes and not be perfect
- protest any treatment from other people that feels bad, disrespectful, or harmful to you
- ask questions when you don't understand
- ask for what you want and need
- negotiate to get things changed
- say no to requests that are unrealistic
- ignore other people's advice

- make your own decisions
- receive recognition for your work and accomplishments
- live and work in a nonabusive environment
- refuse to take responsibility for someone else's problems or pain
- stop trying to mind-read others' needs or wishes

REFERENCES

1. McKay, M., M. Davis, and P. Fanning. 1995. *Messages: The Communication Book.* Oakland, CA: New Harbinger.
2. Foster, D. G., and M. Marshall. 1994. *How Can I Get Through to You?* New York: Hyperion.
3. Clark, C. C. 1996. *Wellness Practitioner: Concepts, Research and Strategies.* New York: Springer.

CHAPTER 8

Success! Keeping the Weight Off for Good: How to Make Your Plan a Permanent Part of Your Life

TIPS FOR MAINTAINING YOUR WEIGHT LOSS

You're losing weight; you're feeling good. Now what? Changing your lifestyle is not always easy, and sticking with these changes can present a challenge. By building in specific checkpoints, you can maintain progress and even increase it. Here are some other ways to maintain your weight loss:

1. Remember to eat slowly and to chew your food well.
2. Avoid serving food family-style. There is too much temptation to overeat.
3. Serve up plates with appropriate portions and avoid asking for seconds.
4. Using smaller plates will make portions look larger.
5. Never eat out of the bag or carton.
6. Ask for half- or smaller portions when eating out or eyeball your appropriate portion, set the rest aside, and ask for a doggie bag right away.
7. Put a note reminding yourself to verify your progress and reward yourself for your excel-

lence on each month's calendar. Appropriate rewards might be an evening to yourself, soaking in a bubble bath and reading a new book, a night out at the movies with your friends while your partner watches the kids, that sweater you've been eyeing in a catalog, or a beautiful basket of fresh fruits.

8. Take regular readings on your feelings and relationships, by taking the "Could Your Relationships Be Hindering Your Weight Loss?" quiz once a month and take steps so that you can answer no to all of the questions.

9. Start small and keep it fun. Taking small steps and being consistent is much better than overreaching and then quitting because you've made it too hard for yourself. To keep it fun, share goals with a friend and agree to meet for herbal tea to check on each other's progress once a week. You'll have time to catch up and keep each other healthy and on target.

10. Keep written records of daily and weekly progress. If you overeat on holidays or other occasions, remind yourself of your progress and encourage yourself to get right back on your lifelong regimen. Remember: everybody makes mistakes. It's no big deal.

11. Use visualization daily to picture yourself successful in taking off weight and keeping it off. Put up pictures of you at your skinniest so that you'll be inspired.

12. Vary foods and exercise so you'll never be bored. Boredom is too good an excuse to quit your program. If you usually walk, ask a friend to take a water aerobics class with you. If you always have orange juice for breakfast, try grapefruit instead. You'll be surprised how lit-

tle changes can make a big difference in your day.

13. Walk, dance, meditate, or listen to calming music during your breaks instead of eating, and find other ways to work exercise and other stress relievers into your daily calendar.

14. Take the stairs whenever you can. Walk to the bus stop rather than taking your car. Mow your own lawn instead of hiring someone.

15. Celebrate anniversaries (week, month, year) of your new lifestyle and tell others about your progress. Be proud of what you've accomplished! You deserve it!

16. Nourish your spirit. Use stress management techniques to relax your mind and keep your spirit at peace. Then you'll be able to make eating and lifestyle decisions that enhance your life.

17. Remind yourself that you've succeeded at things before and you can succeed at this!

BACKSLIDING

Trudy was a thirty-two-year-old mother of two teenage boys. She worked part-time as a nurse at a local health care center. Through hard work, she'd made some important changes in her meal plans and walked two miles every day with a neighbor. Then Trudy had a fight with a coworker who stole her parking place and got a cold. Unfortunately, she didn't stay home and rest, and her cold turned into pneumonia. That kept her from exercising with her neighbor for weeks. At first, Trudy lost weight because she didn't want to eat anything but soup and juice. Then her appetite returned and she ate two peanut butter cookies one of her sons gave her. Before she knew it, she was in the kitchen, binging on the ice cream her husband had promised not to buy.

When you make changes in your life, eat more healthful foods, and start to exercise regularly, you will feel more self-confident, more in control of your life. Everything seems great. All goes well until you meet a high-stress situation, something that threatens your high self-confidence and throws you for a loop.

Backsliding can happen. Trudy's backslide was set up by illness, but it could just as easily be due to a job loss, death in the family, new boss, or any number of high-stress situations. Trudy's stress level was already high, being a parent of two boys who sometimes got into trouble in school when her husband went away on business trips, which he frequently did. The argument with her coworker pushed Trudy's stress level over the edge. She felt the stress of not being sure what to do about her lost parking spot, and her immune system bore the brunt of this stress. Unable to fight off the viruses that are always lurking in our environment, Trudy got sick.

The emotions Trudy felt were triggered by her negative emotions such as her feelings toward the conflict with her coworker and maybe by her resentment at having to raise the boys alone so much of the time. You may be surprised to learn that backsliding can also be triggered by positive emotions like those experienced when getting married or having a child (or grandchild), or at celebrations or other supposedly "happy" situations. Anything that is high-stress, even if it's supposed to be a happy event, can trigger a stress reaction. If you don't have the tools to cope with the situation, you will resort to old behaviors that make you feel better, like eating.

Many overweight people use escape or avoidance to cope with strong feelings. Are you one of those people? If you are, even if you have learned the tools presented in this book, you can still backslide if you feel overwhelmed or if something makes you lose sight of your goal: to lose weight. Once that happens, binge eating can return, along with feelings of helplessness, hopelessness, and giving up. "What's the use?" you may tell yourself. "I can't deal with this. I may as well give up my dream of losing weight."

Now you're feeling vulnerable and are in the perfect mind-set to slip back into old eating patterns. You may even start telling yourself, "I need a reward. I've been so good for so long," or, "That apple pie is going to help me cope with all my stress." If you're in a situation fraught with stress, it's going to be hard to stick to your plan.

Just remember, it's not that bad if you backslide. Don't punish yourself. Don't give up on yourself, either. It's only a temporary slip. You can get back on the plan. Staying positive is the key. If you don't stay positive, you may end up focusing entirely on food and then you may start binging. Tell yourself, "OK, so I slipped. I'll start back on my eating and exercising plan tomorrow [or as soon as you can]. I will not allow myself to get negative and down on me."

High-stress situations can't always be anticipated, but if they can, then anticipate them and take steps to reduce your stress. If they can't and you backslide, just sleep on your actions. Treat yourself with kindness. You deserve it!

Meanwhile, take the following steps to overcome backsliding:

1. **Jot down your favorite excuses for binge eating.** The sooner you confront the ways you sabotage your weight loss plans, the sooner you can control them. Are you the kind of person who says, "My life is so stressful, I don't have time to exercise"? Or maybe you tell yourself, "I worked overtime today; I deserve a big reward." You may even tell yourself you're justified in

eating junk foods because they "calm me down." Whatever excuses you give yourself, pay attention to them and don't let them take hold.

2. **Identify your high-stress situations.** Once you recognize what may trigger backsliding, you are on your way to fixing it. The earlier you can recognize these triggers, the sooner you can take action to reduce your stress. Keep paper clips in chapters 4, 5, and 6 on your favorite stress-reducing food, tool, or exercise and remind yourself to stick with it. You'll not only be proud of yourself; you'll feel more confident and stay on your weight loss path.

3. **Write down an action plan for high-stress situations.** You've identified your high-stress situations. The next step is to have a plan in place. Don't wait until you're being overwhelmed by stress to try to reason it out. That just won't work. When the stress hits it may be too late to find a plan. Choose your plan while you're reasonably relaxed and feel in charge of your life. Write down your favorite positive self-talk phrases and keep them handy. Also keep close at hand your relaxation tapes and whatever other strategies you found in chapter 5 that work for you.

4. **Keep "just one" out of your vocabulary.** Avoid telling yourself, "Just one more cookie," or, "Just one more piece of pie and I'll quit." "Just one"-ing is too hard. Instead, set up situations that are apt to result in positive, not negative, outcomes. Don't have the food around in the first place and don't let other people in the house keep it around you. If they have to have it, let them keep it in their room or locked away someplace you don't know about. Better yet, use the strategies in chapter 7 to get them to

provide support for your weight loss program, including not tempting you. When you want a treat, don't bring the food into the house. Have your taste of your "forbidden foods" at a restaurant in plain view of God and everybody.

5. **Learn to right yourself quickly if you slip.** Sure, it's best not to backslide, but you're human and humans make mistakes. Make a contract with yourself in advance that sets out exactly how much you will allow yourself to eat if you start binging. Keep that contract close at hand, maybe taped to your refrigerator door.

6. **Refuse to berate yourself.** Be positive. Refuse to call yourself names. It won't do any good anyway, and it can do a lot of harm. Always remember to treat yourself gently. You deserve it!

7. **Turn your backsliding into a learning event.** When it's over, ask yourself, "What positive thing did I learn from this?" Maybe it's that you won't let it happen again or that yes, you did binge, but it's fixable as long as you keep believing in yourself.

CHALLENGE YOUR NEGATIVE THINKING

Don't create your own obstacles to weight loss. You need to interrupt any negative thoughts that could lead to backsliding. Look at the following list and see which one of these negative thinking patterns you need to change so you won't backslide:

Jumping to conclusions. Are you the kind of person who assumes something negative is going to happen? Are you sure you know what other people are thinking and it's about you and it's 99 percent negative? Take a break and reason this out. How can you or anyone else know what someone else is thinking? There is no way to do that. If you want to know what someone else is thinking, ask the person. You'll be surprised what he or she tells you. Work from words other people say, not your negative assumptions and self-talk. Your world will be a lot brighter and your reasoning will be, too.

All-or-nothing-at-all thinking. Listen to yourself and ask a trusted friend to remind you when you say things like, "I can't do this," "This will never work," and "Everyone binges." Banish words like *everyone, can't,* and *never* to the wastebasket. They're useless and they only make you feel worse. Challenge yourself with comments like, "What makes me think I can't do this? I've accomplished things before and I can do it now," "This will work, but I have to give it a decent chance," and, "Not everyone binges and I don't have to unless I choose to."

Predicting a bad outcome. Sometimes it's hard not to get into gloom and doom, but you can stay above it. Instead, predict happiness and joy. Talk yourself into having a great time no matter what you're doing. Listen to what you tell yourself and be more positive. Stop yourself in midsentence if you have to, but do it!

Ignoring the good things that happen. Yes, there are many bad things that happen, but guess what? They are usually balanced off with good things if you pay attention. Don't allow yourself to get sucked down into the mire of "nothing good ever happens." Instead, tell yourself, "Look at the whole picture," or, "Put this in perspective." We're not talking about sugarcoating everything, but try to see the full spectrum of reality. Take time to do that. It will be well worth your effort.

Degrading yourself. You are not a bad person. You may have done some things you're not proud of. So has anyone else who is truthful enough to admit it. Don't call yourself names or put yourself down because of it. Vow to do better and just carry on. You'll be fine.

Self-blaming. Stop yourself when you hear, "It's all my fault," and related comments. When stressed, you may feel yourself falling into a self-blaming condition. *Fault* and *blame* are two other words to throw in the wastebasket. They're just not helpful. Take responsibility and carry on. You'll feel a lot better and make a lot more progress.

"Shoulds." Holding the belief that you or someone else must act only one way can set you up for heartbreak and failure. No one, including you, *should* do anything. Sure, many unpleasant and upsetting things happen, but that doesn't mean they should or shouldn't. Our clients sometimes tell us, "My husband shouldn't have brought that layer cake into the house," or, "He should understand me; he's known me long enough to know what I want." "Shoulds" are especially negative patterns. When you hear yourself saying or thinking, "This shouldn't happen to me," rephrase it to, "This is happening and I can deal with it." Or if you hear yourself saying or thinking, "He should understand me," rephrase it to, "I want him to understand, but he can't read my mind, so I'm going to tell him exactly how I feel."

Holding your feelings in. Do you have a difficult time being as direct and honest as you would like? Guess what? You're not alone, but you can learn to speak up. You'll be surprised how much pressure you take off yourself by being honest about your feelings.

Avoiding. Do you try to put things off and bury your head in the sand instead of admitting the obvious? If so, you may be avoiding situations that you need to confront so you can feel better about yourself.

Putting yourself last. It's OK to put yourself last once in a while, but if it's a habitual pattern, it just isn't healthy. Seek balance in all things and vow to put yourself first at least every other time. You deserve it!

Being aggressive. Do you simmer for a long time and then blow up? Do your friends describe you as someone with a temper? It's normal to feel angry and upset when things go wrong, but if you feel angry and resentful all the time and take it out on yourself or others, you're headed down a self-destructive path. Get some help from a counselor.

Being passive. Being submissive is just as unhealthy as being aggressive. Pretending you don't have strong feelings because you don't want to "rock the boat" may lead to more unhappiness than is necessary. By denying yourself your right to be treated with respect, you could end up in an aggressive or abusive relationship. You don't deserve that. Take an assertiveness course or get some counseling.

YOU'RE A SUCCESS

Congratulations! You've worked your way through this book and now you know how to develop the attitude and skills to take off weight and keep it off. You deserve to be the weight that's healthful for you! You'll find that as you work toward your goal, it's getting easier and easier and closer and closer.

Be sure to stick with your plan and don't ever get discouraged. Remember, even if you backslide, you can get back on track and apply what you've learned here. Persevere. You're sure to be successful!

CONTACT DR. CLARK

Carolyn Chambers Clark would like to hear about your weight-loss experiences. She's also interested in hearing your questions, comments, and suggestions for a second edition or a related book.

Please write to her by Earthmail at ~cccwellness @earthlink.net or contact her through her website at *http://home.earthlink.net/~cccwellness.*

Dr. Clark offers workshops, consultation, and retreats based on the principles and practices presented in this book. These programs are appropriate for couples, individuals, health professionals, and others interested in healthy weight loss and other complementary health and wellness practices. If you wish to receive information about these programs please write to her at her e-mail address. Details will be sent to you upon request.

CONTACT DR. ROSCH

Dr. Rosch would also like to hear from you.

Please contact him at stress124@earthlink.net or visit his homepage at www.stress.org.

oats
lima beans
raisins
peas

bananas
mushrooms
cabbage
spinach

---

chicken, spinach
eggs, peas

---

turkey
salmon

---

mackerel
cooked cabbage
bananas +

---

clams, oysters
sardines, crab,
herring

---

fresh dark uncooked
vegetables (green)

---

eggs, broccoli

---

mushrooms, lima beans
yogurt nuts, eggs
oranges, grapefruit, rice

Index

Improve your mood, lose weight
and curb your cravings, simply
by learning the amazing . . .

SECRETS *of* SEROTONIN

CAROL HART

You don't need a prescription for it and you can't buy it at a drug store—that's because serotonin is a natural hormone that you already possess. Now, author Carol Hart tells you how to increase your serotonin levels through food, and exercise, and other natural ways to control your mood swings, your weight, food and alcohol cravings, and much more!

**AVAILABLE WHEREVER BOOKS ARE SOLD
FROM ST. MARTIN'S PAPERBACKS**

SERO 3/98

"GSH IS THE UNSUNG ANTIOXIDANT . . .
IT MAY BE THE ONE THAT MAKES ALL
THE OTHERS WORK. A MUST-READ."
—Bestselling author Robert C. Atkins, M.D.

GLUTATHIONE

The Ultimate Antioxidant

ALAN H. PRESSMAN, D.C., PH.D., C.C.N.
WITH SHEILA BUFF

Everyday life can be toxic to your health—fight back
with GLUTATHIONE, a natural protein considered
to be the king of all antioxidants. Acting as "nature's
policeman," Glutathione rounds up and neutralizes
the toxins that pollute our systems, and may help
battle a wide range of disorders, from allergies to
AIDS, cancer to cataracts, and much, much more!

"Dr. Pressman, in this easily readable book,
provides us with a definitive understanding
of how glutathione works."
—Bestselling author Gary Null

AVAILABLE WHEREVER BOOKS ARE SOLD
FROM ST. MARTIN'S PAPERBACKS

REALIZE THE NATURAL HEALING POTENTIAL OF YOUR BODY.

In his lifetime, spiritual pioneer Edgar Cayce helped
thousands experience the wonders of holistic medicine.
Now, his writings are interpreted and updated by
William McGarey, M.D., a medical doctor who has
used Cayce's methods to heal thousands.

You, too, can learn to understand the secrets of
self-healing, including:

• *Emotional, lifestyle, sleep, and dietary patterns that affect your
body's automatic healing process—and how you can improve them.*
• *How energy medicine can keep you ahead of rising health-care costs.*
• *The importance of aura and energy fields, internal electrical activity,
and homeostasis.* • *Understanding meditation and purification as
tools to energize your spiritual pyramid and encourage your body
to heal.* • *The acid/alkaline balance, its importance, and the
foods you can use to alter it.* • *Stress reduction, dream
interpretation, and past-life therapy.*

HEALING MIRACLES

USING YOUR BODY ENERGIES FOR SPIRITUAL AND PHYSICAL HEALTH

WILLIAM A. MCGAREY, M.D.

AVAILABLE WHEREVER BOOKS ARE SOLD
FROM ST. MARTIN'S PAPERBACKS

DISCOVER THE MEDICAL MIRACLE THAT CAN HALT, REVERSE, AND MAY EVEN <u>CURE</u> OSTEOARTHRITIS

THE ARTHRITIS CURE

After years of suffering from degenerative arthritis, millions of people have finally found relief. Learn the amazing nine-point program outlined in the #1 bestselling ARTHRITIS CURE and discover the safe, natural way—without expensive prescription drugs and without side-effects—to end arthritis suffering once and for all!

"After two months on this remedy…I have stopped limping, I am playing tennis and ice skating with less pain and my knees have stopped swelling."
—Jane Brody's "Personal Health" column in *The New York Times*

THE ARTHRITIS CURE
Jason Theodosakis, M.D., M.S., M.P.H., Brenda Adderly, M.H.A., & Barry Fox, Ph.D.

AVAILABLE WHEREVER BOOKS ARE SOLD
FROM ST. MARTIN'S PRESS

AC 11/98